Metaphysical Secrets
for
Health and Success in Life

Printed by:
InstaBook Maker (tm)

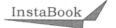

All rights reserved

InstaBooks are distributed and printed through:

INSTABOOK

For more information write to:

InstaBook Corporation
1325 NW 9th Ave
Gainesville, Fl. 32605

www.instabook.net

InstaBook Canada Inc.

30 Community Ave, Unit #2
Stoney Creek, ON
L8E 2Y2

www.instabook.ca

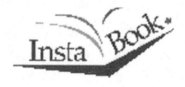

PRINTED AND BOUND IN CANADA

Order this book online at www.trafford.com
or email orders@trafford.com

Most Trafford titles are also available at major online book retailers.

Note for Librarians: A cataloguing record for this book is available from Library
and Archives Canada at www.collectionscanada.ca/amicus/index-e.html

Printed in Victoria, BC, Canada.

ISBN: 978-1-4251-8061-4 (soft)
ISBN: 978-1-4251-8062-1 (ebook)

*We at Trafford believe that it is the responsibility of us all, as both individuals
and corporations, to make choices that are environmentally and socially sound.
You, in turn, are supporting this responsible conduct each time you purchase a
Trafford book, or make use of our publishing services. To find out how you are
helping, please visit www.trafford.com/responsiblepublishing.html*

*Our mission is to efficiently provide the world's finest, most comprehensive
book publishing service, enabling every author to experience success.
To find out how to publish your book, your way, and have it available
worldwide, visit us online at www.trafford.com*

Trafford rev. 5/26/2009

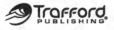 www.trafford.com

North America & international
toll-free: 1 888 232 4444 (USA & Canada)
phone: 250 383 6864 ♦ fax: 250 383 6804 ♦ email: info@trafford.com

The United Kingdom & Europe
phone: +44 (0)1865 487 395 ♦ local rate: 0845 230 9601
facsimile: +44 (0)1865 481 507 ♦ email: info.uk@trafford.com

10 9 8 7 6 5 4 3 2 1

Table of Contents

Introduction

At one time or another we have wondered, how does the World really work? Scientists tell us one thing and religious leaders tell us something totally different. This text has been written to bridge the gap between the elusive world of mysticism and the concrete world of hard science.

In this book, you will find that the light of knowledge uncovers many shrouded methods of healing. You will find plausible technical answers and techniques you can use to influence the subtle sea of energy fields that we live in. Many of the techniques in this book should be considered as basics of life that everyone should know and use. For the first time, the basics of Metaphysics are written in an easy-to-read, how-to format for everyone to enjoy,

Although there are references to various religions, this book is not meant to be a religious text. The ideas portrayed are to be considered as 'How-to-dos based on observation and experiment' and not by any theological values. You will come across many things that ring that familiar 'wow' in you, and will want to refer to those ideas later. I suggest that as you read this book, you underline or highlight items of interest for your future reference.

The knowledge contained in this text can be one of the most powerful tools you will find for the living of a truly successful and healthy lifestyle. The conceptual truths of life contained in this volume are truly building blocks on how the subtle energies about us influence and control our lives.

If you want to make personal breakthroughs in health and successful living, this book is a must to read. Chapter by chapter you will find techniques you can use immediately to change your life. At this point, all that is left to be said is to turn the pages, read, and be challenged.

Raymond T. Kranyak, Ph.D.

Acknowledgements

This book is based on many years of study on scientific fact, religious beliefs, and healing methodologies. As I journeyed through life there were some unexplainable things that I experienced on a regular basis that led me into study and research in the field of Psychic Energy.

I am greatly indebted to the many researchers, lecturers, and practitioners of the psychic, metaphysical, martial arts, and philosophy, without whom, I could not have gained the spark of knowledge that started me down the path of metaphysics, first as a student and then as a teacher and researcher.

My final thanks go to those who presently and in the future will continue to keep working on and expanding the knowledge of metaphysics. It is only our better understanding of the unchanging universal laws interaction with the world and various religions that will allow humanity to evolve to higher physical and spiritual levels.

What Is Metaphysics?

History of Metaphysics

Metaphysics has been around for centuries, but today we still have not really established whether Metaphysics is a moral code of ethics, a religion, a philosophy, an occultism, or a science.

Metaphysics has been considered a branch of philosophy devoted to the examination of the nature of reality, specifically the relationship between mind and matter. Metaphysics also raises speculation upon unanswerable questions that elude analysis, scientific observation, or experimentation.

The word metaphysics came as a result of the writings of Aristotle. Aristotle was a master of philosophy in 384-322 B.C., who presented what he called the First Philosophy after Physics. Aristotle is considered to be the father of metaphysics. In the Greek language the result was '**meta-physic**' which meant '**after physics**'. Metaphysical systems in the history of philosophy started with Aristotle's thoughts. Since then, Descartes and Spinoza expounded upon the subject. Since the mid-19th century, philosophy has for the most part denied any validity to metaphysical thought. Modern interest in metaphysics has centred on analyzing the thought-provoking metaphysical statements of the past.

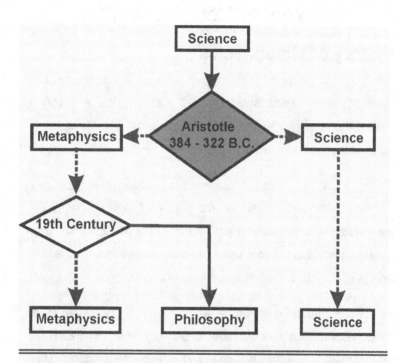

Figure 1.1 The Emergence of Metaphysics

Metaphysics has been described as occultism, mysticism, transcendentalism, mystical interpretation, cabalism, reincarnationism, yogism, hyperphysics, supernaturalism, psychicism, pseudopsychology, a secret art, an esoteric science, the study of occult lore, alchemy, astrology, psychometry, spiritualism, magic, sorcery, fortune-telling, crystal-gazing, palmistry, clairvoyance, second sight, animal magnetism, mesmerism, hypnotism, hypnotic trance, and probably anything else that man can dream up without an explanation.

Personally, I think that Metaphysics is a personal belief structure developed over time based on one's theories of expertise. Metaphysics influences everything in our life from religious to scientific beliefs.

Most people have no problem with debating metaphysical thoughts on the subject of religious beliefs. But you will find those very same people will usually shy away from the discussion of metaphysical thoughts in the realm of scientific beliefs. The thought that science is only a collection of beliefs based on observation brings the same type of religious outcry of heresy from those dedicated people of the scientific community. Scientists believe that they work in a science-driven world composed of solid facts.

Science is based on observing facts as a structure of the scientific discipline. These facts are also based on belief in the accuracy of the scientific method. This methodology perpetuates itself by the belief that it is the only way to distinguish true facts. Thus the scientific method is composed of the belief that the facts that are repetitively observable must be true. Such a structure of facts assembled through this methodology has in the past rendered such proven fact as 'the Earth is flat'. Since then we have found that the Earth is round or, as most recently discovered, slightly pear-shaped. At one time there was a scientific fact that stated 'man will disintegrate if he surpasses the maximum velocity of 30 miles per hour'. Since then humankind has broken the sound barrier, which at one time was also considered unbreakable. We also believed the statement that 'if man was meant to fly, he would have wings like a bird'. Today humankind flies everywhere on our Earth as well as out of the Earth's protective atmosphere. A long standing medical fact was that 'if a runner attempts to break the four-minute mile, the strain on his body will cause his heart to burst'. Today, the basic standard for an Olympic competitor is not whether or not they can break the four-minute mile, but by how much!

These outdated quotes, as well as many more that you can think of, were based on scientific facts derived using the method of scientific observation. The people who broke these barriers for humankind were individuals who stepped away from the known facts and used metaphysical thought, which led them and the world into a new reality. These leaders changed the scientifically proven impossibilities into the realities of the world that we enjoy today.

This is why I suggest that science is just a structure of beliefs that are based on observation using today's most sophisticated scientific instruments. Tomorrow we will have more sophisticated scientific methods and instruments that will cause today's scientific beliefs to vanish without a trace. Tomorrow we will have a new set of facts to look at, and as a result our scientific beliefs will change. Science is important and is needed to validate that we are actually advancing as a civilization. But in the right perspective, science is useful but cannot presently venture in to the metaphysical field with certainty and accuracy.

This is where metaphysics starts to cross into the scientific realm, even if our friends in the white lab coats disagree.

Metaphysics is the study of life about us. We learn from previously documented metaphysical and scientific knowledge which was based on observation. We add to this pool of knowledge with new observations created by our life experience.

In metaphysics there is no one great truth but a series of beliefs that each one of us puts together based on the many truths that we observe and experience in our lifetime.

Many students of philosophy ask the question, 'Will the content of Metaphysics change through time?' My answer is 'yes'. When we first studied metaphysics, humankind set down a series of universal truths based on our understandings of that time. Many of these truths have been rewritten through the centuries as our understanding of the universe and humankind evolved. The same basic truths in metaphysics are still as sound as they were at the time of their inception. The difference is that through the gaining of more knowledge we have been better able to define these truths. We will continue to redefine the truths of metaphysics until all of the non-understandable things of life are understood and used by everyone. As we learn to better define metaphysical ideas, we will come closer to knowing the truth and meaning of our existence.

Realms of Existence

Levels of Existence

Metaphysics is not just a realm of beliefs within itself. Some of the principles of Metaphysics also show up in the ancient Sanskrit scrolls and can be compared to the seven principles or seven levels of existence. Most of our civilization lives on the first realm of existence, and few individuals venture to the second realm of existence; even fewer achieve the up to the fifth realm of existence. Only a few exercise the sixth and seventh realms of existence. Not everyone seeks to follow the spiritual path, and these individuals may be satisfied to live their life in the one or two realms which they choose.

The Planes of Existence

7. Spiritual Existence

6. Spiritual Plane

5. Intuitive Existence

4. Energy Plane

3. Astral Plane

2. Intellectual Existence

1. Physical Plane

As you notice, some of the levels are named as planes of existence and others are named as types of existence. This is not an error. The planes of existence are named so as they are skills that one can learn and use in life. Early humankind existed as groups of hunting tribes. As hunting was the major aspect of existence, this indicates humankind operated in the physical plane as hunting is considered to be one of the levels within the physical plane.

The Physical Plane

The entire world we live in operates within the physical plane of existence, as we require using these basic skills for day-to-day survival. People who spend all of their time in the physical plane of existence follow the rituals of acquiring wealth and fulfilling all of their physical desires. Their thoughts seldom go beyond that realm. The physical plane is where they find their total personal satisfaction. If you are alive and reading this book, you probably have a good handle on the mastery of the physical plane. There is one catch to the physical plane, and that is that we are in this life that is governed by the physical plane for only a short period of time. The mastery of this plane is good only for the physical lifetime you are in. When you move on from this life to a spiritual realm of the great beyond, the physical skills will then be of no real value. If you return for another lifetime, you will be required to relearn and again master the survival elements of the physical plane before working on achieving that lifetime's purpose.

Intellectual Existence

The people who occupy the intellectual level may or may not have mastered the physical or any other plane of existence. These individuals make the assumption that knowledge is power. They spend their lives studying and collecting knowledge. Many people on the intellectual plane have mastered the ability to collect knowledge. However, many of the people in this plane may never put to use the knowledge that they collect in their lifetime. Those who choose to live in this plane alone find that the collecting of knowledge and knowing many things can be very self-satisfying. They may not learn that collecting knowledge without using it is a means to no end. It is only when the knowledge learned is used in any or all of the other planes or realms that it holds any value to its keeper. The collection of knowledge, whether it is through reading, learning in classes, or experiencing in life is a critical element to mastering any or all planes of existence. But beware that the collection of knowledge by itself masters nothing.

I would like to challenge you on that thought of 'knowledge is power'. I would like to suggest that the real power is in putting the knowledge to good use.

Astral Plane

At one time or another everyone experiences a step into the astral plane. This can be as a dream or, at the other end of the spectrum, a step into another time and place without your physical body. The people that are in the astral realm are known as the dreamers, and for some reason or other they operate in a totally different reality. These people usually have mastered the advanced use of their imagination. We most frequently use our imagination for daydreaming and other non-productive flights of fancy. However, through the conscious use of the imagination, we can see well beyond the physical plane by breaking the physical realm's barriers of time, distance, and solidity. Imagination is the tool of the astral plane and, once mastered, it can allow you to see distant physical locations, the past, the future, and assist you in solving any problem. This is the plane of the seers of the future.

Energy Plane

The energy plane is probably one of the most controversial planes that humankind will encounter. It is in this plane that we can feel and experience the sea of psychic energy. Universal psychic energy is difficult to measure by any means except by the use of physical feelings. The energy plane is where the healers of today reside. These are the people who have developed their imagination to the point where they can manipulate the energy field around them to assist in the healing of their selves and others. The energy plane can be used to manipulate matter, protect you from the negative energy of the surroundings, or make the future that you wish to see come to pass today. The energy plane is as important to health as the physical plane is to our existence in the physical life.

Intuitive Existence

The intuitive existence is where many people that have mastered the physical, astral, and energy planes of existence choose to reside. This plane is where mastery of our existence on this Earth is recognized and we choose to use the skills that we have mastered in the physical, astral, and energy planes to either live a comfortable life or share what we know with humankind. Many of the richest people and the world's great leaders have mastered these planes to enjoy an intuitive existence. These are the people who have hunches that they use to gain success in achieving their desired goals in life. People operating at this level instinctively avoid things that will give them problems and work on things that will bring them success in this life. Those who have achieved this level of existence can choose to live a comfortable life and just seem to have what they need come their way.

Operating your life at this level definitely has many advantages over the mere existence on the endless treadmill that many souls have chosen to monotonously plod through in this life.

Spiritual Plane

Life on this plane has a distinctly different pursuit. The mastery of the other realms is not important to the occupants of this plane. The main goal of the people on the spiritual plane is to gain spiritual knowledge and experience. The people in this realm can tell you of all of the major religions of the world but may not possess the ability to drive an automobile, as this mode of transportation is just not important to them. One of the differences that distinguish the person operating in this plane from the person living in the knowledge realm is that the person in the spiritual plane seeks only spiritual and religious knowledge. Usually the goal of someone living in this realm is to gain the knowledge that can lead to a spiritual existence in preparation for the life beyond the grave. The people on this path can be seekers of a particular spiritual knowledge as well as being masters of various spiritual and religious principles.

Spiritual Existence

Many people wish to achieve this level of existence but are not willing to put in the work or they lack the discipline required to achieve the spiritual existence. When a person operates in the spiritual level of existence, their decisions are based on doing what is required for the good of humankind or to maintain a universal truth. These people are usually very accomplished and have all of their needs met. Usually their needs are few, and they enjoy a modest but comfortable lifestyle.

When a person living in a spiritual existence has a need, it appears to magically be fulfilled without having to work for it. As they are working on maintaining the greater truths of the universe, the universe responds by fulfilling their personal needs so that they can continue in the great work unhampered by the needs of the physical plane. People that operate at this level may appear to have mastery in any realm that they enter, but in reality they do not. Because their focus is always on the universal greater good, their decisions are usually easier to make and the solutions to the problem are easier to put in motion.

The greatest skill used in the spiritual existence is the ability to influence others to make changes that will influence the greater good for all. To live within this realm is really to be in this world but not a part of it.

Which Plane or Existence are You in?

Most of our philosophers have the idea that the universe operates in a series of steps. Steps or levels of achievement are really a thought restriction that we put upon ourselves in the human existence. Many of us have a belief structure that leads us to feel that we have to master one level before moving up to the next level. Upon achieving the entry level, we believe that we must move up to the intermediate level, then to the advanced level, and finally to the mastery level of a subject. We are trained to think according to this linear achievement concept by our school system. We all know that to be in 'grade 2' you must master 'grade 1'. To move to 'grade 3' you must master 'grade 2'. This model for doing things works in the school system as a way to teach and measure scholastic ability. Because our society has trained us that life operates this way in the school system, we assume that everything in the universe operates according to this same method of steps of achievement. I would like to suggest that this is not how things in the universe actually work.

If we are governed by levels of achievement, then it goes without saying that to achieve the gold medal at the Olympics you must first study physical education to know how to become the best athlete. The basics required would be graduating from high school, then to graduating with honours in physical education from a college or university, then getting a Master's degree and Doctorate in physical education before you can compete at the Olympics, alone hope to win the gold medal. This is the fallacy of step thinking.

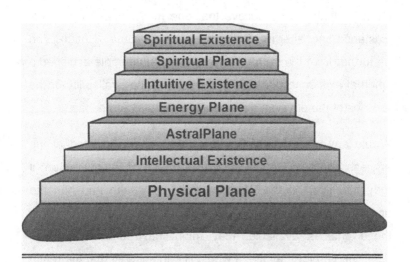

Figure 2.1 The Assumed Steps of Enlightenment

For someone to be a gold medallist runner, the only requirement is to run faster than everyone else that you compete against. There are no complicated educational requirements; there are no steps to achievement; all there is, is to enter the Olympic tryouts and run faster than everyone else that entered. As long as you can outrun the other contestants in all the races, you can win the gold medal. You may not even be able to read or write, but if you can run, you can win the gold medal. If you wish to master something in this life, all you have to do is to study and practice what you wish to master until you gain the mastery of that thing.

By step thinking, we believe that one may achieve a spiritual existence only after mastering the physical plane. Nothing can be further from the truth. Many very spiritual people achieved a spiritual existence because of the lack of the availability of the luxuries of the physical plane, such as wealth and riches.

Would any of our great Eastern philosophers have spent the endless hours of life following the pursuit of enlightenment if they had lived in the Western world of wealth and had the opportunity of operating a business for personal gain? With these choices available, they might have chosen a much different path for their life. I would like to suggest that the realm you choose to master in this life is based on choices and is not a hierarchy of achievement.

Just think of how many things for which we see a series of steps to achievement, where there are no steps of achievement except the ones that we construct in our minds. With this thought in mind, let us look again at the levels of achievement, not as a series of steps but as a number of distinctly different realms that we choose to live in to master. A person who chooses to live in the physical plane and master it is no less of a person than the person who chooses to live the spiritual existence and master that. The realm choices we make are based on what we wish to experience in this life. We live and learn by experiencing what is in the realm that we choose.

There are really no steps to mastery of life. Rather, we have to choose which realms we wish to master and live within. A person is not held captive in the physical plane by a lack of personal growth, but stays there as a matter of choice.

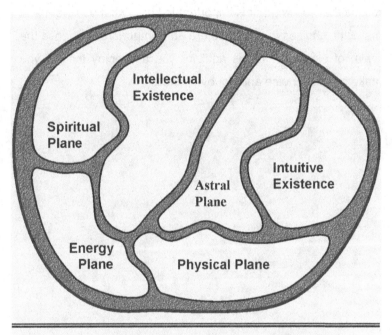

Figure 2.2 The intermingled Planes of Existence

With this knowledge of the planes of existence, a person becomes free to choose the plane of existence that they wish to live in. They make this their personal realm of existence to enjoy and master. Remember that in the universe there are no wrong choices, as you can decide to live as you wish. There are no wrong choices, but there are results that you will ensure from the decisions you make. Make choices that will give you the results that you wish to achieve. If you make a choice that gives undesired results, just decide on another way to get the results that you want. It is important to know what you want and make the choices to get you there. It is important to choose the realm of existence that is right for you and enjoy the life you make by your choice and not by chance.

Your Personal Map of the Universe

History of Mapping

Whether you know it or not, within yourself you carry a personal map of the universe. You started drawing this map in your mind the day that you were born. As you gained experience in life you revised this internal map so you can continually decipher how the universe operates. You will either consciously or unconsciously update this map until the day that you die. This map that you carry within you is a basic tool for survival.

This internal map is made up of your collection of thoughts of how you consider the way things are. This map of the universe is what you constantly mentally refer to so that you can maintain stability and sanity in your life. Without a unique personal mental map of the universe, you would lack having stable points from which to measure reality. The success and satisfaction that you will achieve in life are of a result of how you have set up and managed your map of the universe. If you maintain an accurate mental map of the universe, you will get good results in life. This is the result of making good decisions from a map containing good information. If you have a poorly assembled map of the universe, you will get poor results. The mental institutions are filled with people who have inaccurate maps of the universe within themselves. Their maps are so far removed from the actual way the universe operates that they have no reference to reality and require special assistance to survive in a way that they will not harm themselves or others.

As human beings, we constantly refer to our map of the universe. As we learn new things, we add them to our map. Our map is made up not only of personal beliefs but of scientific facts and any other knowledge that we have reaped since birth. Some of the information in our universal maps could be the way to get to work or school, how to cook supper, how to treat others, one's religious beliefs, one's work ethics, etc. The list goes on and on, comprised of all of the knowledge that we have gathered in this lifetime.

Our map of the universe works much like the paper travel maps of the early ocean explorers. In early years of sailing, it was a known fact that the Earth was flat. At that time it was surmised that the Earth was flat because if it was not flat, people would slide to the edge and fall off. Also because the Earth was considered flat, it was believed that if you went too close to the edge, you would indeed fall off of the Earth. At that time, relatively small amounts of the world had been discovered and mapped on a flat piece of parchment. This left the natural assumption that if the Earth could be drawn on a two-dimensional flat piece of parchment, then the Earth was indeed flat.

Explorers, who disappeared, never to return, were assumed to have ventured too close to the edge of the flat Earth and fallen off. As more exploration of the world was done, the maps improved until there was enough knowledge documented for Columbus to surmise that the Earth is not flat, but indeed round.

As humankind through the centuries travelled around the globe, we discovered that if you travel in a direction long enough that you will end up at the exact point at which you started. Our travels into space further confirmed through observation that the Earth is slightly pear-shaped. As humankind explored the Earth and revised the travel maps, our concept of the Earth's shape became more accurate. The Earth, which was previously known to be flat, eventually came to be known as three dimensional in globe shape. As a result, our world travel maps have been revised to show this knowledge in the form of world globes.

Universal Maps

Our internal universal maps work exactly the same way as a travel map. Our ideas of how the Universe we live in operates are based on our personal internal maps. As the early explorers constructed travel maps, our internal universal map is constructed from our collection of life experiences. As we gain additional knowledge through experience, we then edit and add this information to our personal map of the universe. The more information that that we have on our personal map, the greater ability we have to make better decisions in life. By consciously developing and maintaining an accurate universal map we can again have more information to make better decisions.

One of the pitfalls that humankind runs into is that one day in our life many of us decide that our personal map of the universe is the way things are, and we stop revising our map to reflect the changes in the world about us. By falling into that trap, we can spend more time defending our outdated map than learning how the World has changed. When this happens to someone, the defending of an inaccurate personal Universal Map can become a life goal that can eventually cause that individual to slip out of the reality of how things really are. You can find in any old age home individuals who will gladly advise you how to be successful in life based on their outdated universal maps. The problem is that they now are confined to an old age home and have not revised their map since the day they arrived. Their stories make wonderful history lessons from their personal perspective, as an old book would give an insight to a different era. However, realise that the information they freely give is as outdated as their personal universal maps and may not apply to the world as it operates today.

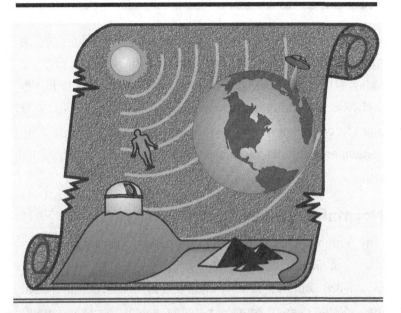

Figure 3.1 Have You examined Your Map of the Universe?

To enjoy a fulfilling life, we must constantly be open to evaluating new ideas and ready to revise our personal maps whenever needed. One of the keys to a happy and successful existence is to have and use an accurate universal map.

As shown in the illustration in Figure 3.1, a universal map contains physical locations of things in the same way a travel map does. The universal map also contains personal beliefs, how you respond to people, how you expect people to treat you, as well as anything that you have experienced in life. In some cases it has been found that some people's maps may contain some information from past lives. If this information is found to be within you, you must realise that the information may be outdated and not applicable to the life that you live today. This information can be in the form of phobias or health problems that you have from an unknown source. These items need to be reviewed and revised so that you can live this life unhampered by this information that may be inappropriate for today.

Normal Mapping Cycle

The normal cycle of operation of a person's Universal Map is shown in Figure 3.2. In life, when we are faced with an experience, our mind will evaluate and revise our universal map. In the case of items of personal safety, this is important. When a small child is learning to walk, the child is working on limited universal map information. When a child has the experience of falling down, immediately the child's universal map is checked and a response is activated based on the severity of the fall. In this case, the response is to revise the universal map. If there was no injury, the universal map is revised to add the ability to walk information. If the child is injured, the response invoked is to revise the universal map to not do that motion again. The result is a revision to the universal map. This repetitive cycle runs within us constantly. This is how humankind learns.

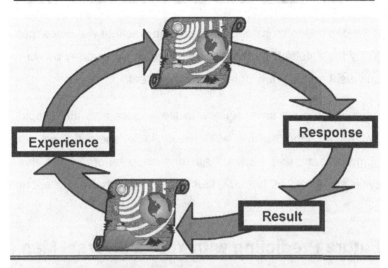

Figure 3.2 The common use of the Universal Map

As we amass information, the cycle works a little differently. We refer to our universal map to make decisions. This second mode of universal map usage is in place when we are not in learning mode. An example of this universal map information mode can be seen when we cross a street. We invoke an experience by looking down the street and observing a fast-moving automobile. Our mind checks our universal map and decides on the speed of the automobile and the past knowledge of success of crossing the road without being hit. Based on this information, our mind invokes a response to wait until the vehicle passes and then to cross the street. This gives us a favourable response which is then added to our universal map as additional information on how to cross the street safely.

If we decided to cross and the response was that we almost got hit by the automobile, then the result would be an entry into our universal map on how not to cross the street.

Anything that we have learned in life is based on this simple cycle. As long as this adaptive cycle is operating, we as humans learn and evolve. As mentioned before, when this cycle stops, we as humans loose touch with the reality about us.

Future Predicting with Your Universal Map

Many of us use our universal map as a collection of all of our past knowledge and really never learn how to unlock the true power of our universal map. Using our universal map effectively can bring us untold success in life. Our universal map can also be used to map the future as easily as mapping our past experiences.

When we use a travel map to choose a trip route, we look for recognizable road names to determine where we are along the trip. If we are lucky enough to get a marked-up travel map from someone who has previously visited our chosen destination, we will have an easier trip. By examining this map, you can see the previously planned trip and notes taken along the way that add to the travel map information. If you are lucky, you may even find a plotted line that will be the guide for your future trip with rest stops added.

When planning a trip, we can choose to either draw a map or mark up a travel map of the route we will take to get to our desired destination. We do this because if we do not know where we are going, how will we ever know when we reach our destination? Do we travel the world and get to our destination by chance or by choice? When physically travelling to a destination in this world, we choose where we want to go, map a route, make plans, and when all preparations are complete, we make the trip.

In travelling there are some basics we follow. The first is to choose a destination. If we do not know where we are going, how will we know when we get there? The second step is to choose the route that we will take. If we do not know the route, we can drive forever and never reach our destination. Then we must decide on the mode of transportation. Will we ride a bicycle, ride a bus, take a train, or drive a car? If the trip is going to be longer than one day, where will we sleep over? For a successful trip, there are many items that have to be attended to.

Future Sketching on Your Universal Map

In life, we can use our universal map to plot our future in the same way as we plot a trip on a travel map. Many of us have been letting our universal map direct where we will go based on our past life experiences without any conscious input. Some of the entries on our universal map are important to keep us safe from personal injury based on experience entries, while other entries can restrict our progress in life.

When we have an experience in life, the experience is entered in our universal map. Our universal map is a collection of the things that we have experienced in our journey through life. When we are faced with an experience that is similar to one previously logged in our universal map, our mind quickly reviews our map and sets in motion a response to the current situation based on the experience logged in our universal map. In the case of personal safety, such as avoiding an oncoming vehicle because your personal map tells you that if you stay there you will get injured, the personal map is very helpful. You will not be injured, and this experience of successfully avoiding an oncoming vehicle will be added to your personal map for future use.

In some cases, you can have areas in your universal map that have become obsolete or were unconsciously written when you were too young to make an accurate assessment of the situation. An example of this can be a condition where an individual gains an irrational response to authority. In this case, the person afflicted would have to review their response to authority figures in their universal map, and then do some research into alternate methods of responding to people in authority. The next step would be to set a plan in place for reacting to persons of authority in the future and follow that plan until the desired results are achieved. They may have to revise this plan a few times until their personal universal map guides them to the results that they wish to achieve. Revising your universal map is one of the most powerful things that you can do to live a more vibrant life.

If you can change the way you respond to life by revising your universal map, you are actually changing the way you will act in the future. Change the way that you will act in the future, and you will change the results that you will get in the future. By changing your future responses in life, you are actually changing your future, as the world will also respond differently to your future responses. This is a very powerful thought, because the only thing we can actually change in life is the way that we respond to an event at any moment in time. By preparing our universal map so that we can respond in a more powerful way when that moment comes is the only way that we can control our destinies.

It is important to note that we can use only the moment of time that we are currently living in. We have no control of any moment of time once it is used up and passes into history.

Dwelling on past moments of time may be nostalgic, but it does not change our current situation. Once a moment of time moves into history, we have no more power to change that moment. What is done is done.

We can not control future moments of time because they can come to pass in a way that we may not suspect. Future moments of time are in a flexible state until they become fixed in the present moment that we live in. The only way that we can exercise control over future events is to prepare for them by plotting how we wish to use our moments in time today in order to take us down the path to the future we wish to live in. The time we use in revising our universal map to prepare for these upcoming situations pays off in our better handling of life's events when we have the opportunity to control the situation in the present. By using this methodology, we can control life's situations and thus build a more powerful personal universal map to live from.

We have just touched on the possibilities available by using our universal map to plot future event responses. In life, actively managing our universal map is the most powerful thing we can do. If we plot how we will respond to future events, the world will reciprocate by responding in a different manner to the situation. When we effectively use mapping to better manage our moments in time, life will give us more favourable results.

If we expand this thought a little further, it is easy to see how we can use our universal map to plot our future in the same manner that we use a road map to plot our journey to a destination. On the road map, we select a time and place where we want to be in the future, we calculate the route, to be taken and estimate when we will leave for the destination. Using the same technique, you can select the home you want to live in, select the type of people you wish to associate with, and select the career that you want. By selecting one of these examples or any other goal you wish to achieve, you will have set a destination to travel to through the time that we are living in. Map out the way you want things to be in your life, and then set a date of when you want it to happen.

The next step is the same as using a road map to plot how you will get to that moment in time with the situation that you have chosen. To reach the destination in the time that you planned and to have everything in place to make the circumstances of that lifestyle come to fruition, what do you have to do?

If you to have a beautiful home, what financial resources do you require? What career does your vision show that supports this lifestyle? What education or training do you need for that career? What does a person like you do to support that lifestyle? When you ask yourself these questions, you are actually mapping the path into the future that will lead you to the lifestyle that you desire.

Once you have mapped the lifestyle that you wish to have, the next step is the one that actually starts to bring the desired lifestyle into the physical realm. Draw the map to your future on a piece of paper. Just as you would refer to a roadmap on your journey to a destination, you must use a paper copy of the journey that you have picked in this physical life as a reference to keep you on track toward your envisioned destination. Refer to your paper map on a daily basis to ensure that you are continuing on the path that you have chosen to travel.

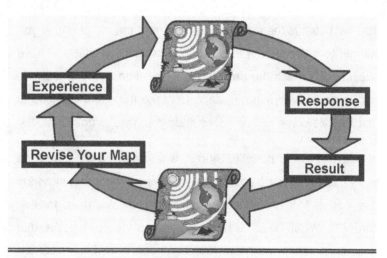

Figure 3.3 Universal Map revising for better Life Results

As you refer to the map, decide what you will do today to take you closer to your envisioned destination in life. For example, if training is needed to move you into a career, what can you do today as a step to get the training? Then do it. If, for example, a sum of money is needed, what can you do today to achieve acquiring that sum of money? Start a savings and investment plan? Just keep referring to your paper map and asking the 'what can I do now?' question until you reach the point of doing something to move down the road to your mapped future. If you do not reach the point of something that you can do right now to make that future happen, you have not asked the question enough times. There is always something that you can do now to move you down the path to your desired future.

Once you have mapped your future, just keep asking yourself the same question over again. What can I do right now to bring me to the lifestyle that I desire? Then tackle that step. By following this methodology, your universal map can be used to actually predict and mould your future.

You may ask, what if ...... , as I am travelling down the road toward my initial vision of my perfect lifestyle, I see a different lifestyle that I wish to pursue? The answer is simple; you made the first paper map of the future lifestyle that you desired. You now can, at any time, either revise that map or draw a new map of the lifestyle that you now desire. As we grow and personally develop, it is not uncommon to make new choices in life based on our expanded knowledge. The important point to remember is to map your future so that you can choose where your life destinations will be. If you do not map your future, you will likely end up somewhere you neither planned for nor wanted.

Your universal map will operate whether you take an interest in using, or not. I would like to encourage you to actively use your universal map as a tool to bring to fruition a glorious life.

How Close Are You to Being a Genius?

The important part of revising and updating personal maps is to understand that using knowledge works in an exponential way. That means that with every new piece of knowledge you attain, there comes the capacity to learn two additional items of knowledge based on the one original one. The knowledge gained by learning the two pieces gives you the ability to expand your knowledge pool by four items based on the learning of the two items of knowledge. The four items of knowledge now give you the ability to learn 16 new items. The next level of ability is to learn 256 new items based on the 16 items. As you can see, it takes very little effort to bring your learning potential into an infinite level of measurement. You may be closer than you imagine to working at the level of a genius. By consciously referring to and updating your personal map of the universe, you can easily achieve a genius level of thinking and achieving. Genius level thinking is simple to achieve and easy to maintain. The ability to operate at a genius level is simply based on the amount of knowledge that you collect, use, and actively manage on your personal map.

We usually define things in a step thinking mode, feeling that one thing has to be achieved before moving to the next. Unfortunately, our brains do not as a rule function in a step mode when we analyze problems. If our brains worked in a step mode, we would never experience moments of stray thoughts as our brain searches for solutions to a problem. When we study one piece of information, our brains can usually find at least two alternate solutions to a single problem. It is harder to find the first solution to a problem than it is to gain the next four or more alternate solutions. Once the exponential operation of our brain finds the first idea, it quickly starts to generate two more ideas. Then the motion is set in place to find at least four or more other viable options to the solution of any problem. When you are looking for a solution to a problem, continue on from the first idea until you find at least four alternatives to consider for the final solution. The block that a number of people have is to stop at the first solution, which in many cases may not be the best solution. A good rule of thumb is that if you have one solution, hold out for at least four other solutions to compare it with.

You are What You Read

Due to the unique exponential operation of our brain, reading is a powerful tool that we can use for tremendous mental capacity expansion. This is why the old adage 'read to become successful' is so true. The more information you gather, the more bits of knowledge you have available to draw from for solutions to problems in life. If you read two books, the knowledge expansion due to the intermingling of information is actually the equivalent of reading four books. How many books have you read today, this week, this year?

Any information that you gather is automatically stored in your personal map of the universe. The quality of the information that you collect is important to your success in this life. If you choose to gather soap opera information and fiction novel information, you will be fashioning your internal map of the universe to the standards of fiction and an entertainment level of reality. Do you really want to relate your real life events as Donny did in the soap opera? Base your personal map on fiction and you will achieve fictional results in life. The quality of your personal universal map is based on the quality of information you put into it. The exponential thinking factor based on fiction novels could give you some interesting information to make life decisions by. Your mind processes information much like a computer. Computers follow the **GIGO** principle. That is 'Garbage In' gives you 'Garbage Out'. Be careful of what you study, your entertainment options, and the people that you associate with. Today's entertainment scripts can be mentally inserted into your map of the universe as tomorrow's decision-making guideposts.

All it takes to unleash your genius potential is to gather good information, evaluate that information, and make conscious decisions based on that knowledge. Keep in mind that every time that you double the information you have, you in fact have squared your idea potential. My only question to you is how many times do you have to double the information in your personal universal map to work at a genius level?

Dreams and Action

Before leaving this section on your universal map there is one precaution to be aware of. That is, you can plot the best universal map that ever existed, but if all you do is map information and never use it in the physical realm, the information will stay in the world of dreams as a dream. It was once said that 'faith without works is dead'. This simple biblical statement simply means that you can believe something is going to happen as much as you want, but if you are unwilling to do something in the physical world to bring it into existence, it will never happen. Reviewing your universal map on a regular basis will help build internal desire and circumstances for you to

get what you want, but only taking the physical action required
will bring your desires to fruition.

Levels of Consciousness

Two Minds

How you live your life is dependent upon the mental level of consciousness in which that you operate. Most people spend their lives reacting to events, laboriously thinking their way through problems. They get results that work, but the effort that they expend to attain these results is far beyond what is required. For the most part, people ignore their intuition and miss many accurate hunches or insights that could make life easier and more productive. Much is known and written about the conscious and subconscious minds. Most people still have reservations about conscious use of their subconscious mind, their most powerful mental faculty.

The human mind is divided into two distinctive parts, the conscious mind' and the subconscious mind. We constantly access the conscious mind and use it to do things such as writing, talking, and actively thinking about a specific subject. The conscious mind is the part of our mind where the ego lives. The ego is simply who we think we are as a person. The conscious mind is the part of our mind that we can very easily control. However, the conscious mind comprises only 10% of our mental abilities. Our usual lack of use of the subconscious mind may be due to ego's wish to have the final say in decisions based on the premises by which we see ourselves.

This way of thinking keeps many of us from recognizing and using the abilities stored in the much more expansive subconscious part of our mind.

Hidden Mental Power

Our subconscious mind is very similar to the iceberg that sank the great ship, Titanic. A contributing factor to the Titanic disaster was the fact that the amount of ice that was visible above water was relatively small. As a matter of fact, only 10% of an iceberg is visible while the other 90% is hidden below the water. The unseen 90% of the iceberg was what cut into the hull and sank the Titanic. The same holds true for our subconscious mind; it is the unseen power source of our mind. The subconscious mind is where 90% of our mental capacity resides.

One of the subconscious mind's functions is to control all of our involuntary body operations such as our heartbeat, breathing, and blood flow, to name just a few. If we did not have a subconscious mind, to remain alive would be a tremendous task. The conscious mind would have to activate every heartbeat, orchestrate every breath, and keep track of all the veins and arteries to ensure that blood would flow to every part of the body. Nature's solution was to hand these functions over to the subconscious mind. The subconscious mind's control over the body's autonomic functions allows the conscious mind

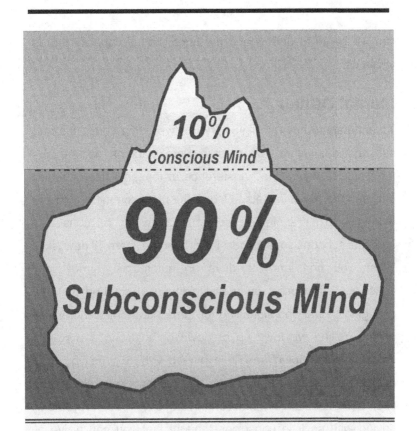

Figure 4.1 The 'Subconscious Mind's' unseen power

to be available for free conscious thought. Even though the subconscious mind controls the autonomic body functions, it is possible, through specialized training, to control body temperature and heartbeat pace by linking the conscious mind to the subconscious mind. Only by personally identifying this link between the conscious mind and the subconscious mind can we begin to understand the huge mental capacity that is within us.

Mental Duties

To understand how the link works between the conscious and subconscious minds, we must explore common occurrences from our life where the transference of thoughts has occurred between the two mindsets. One of the most common mind link examples of a transfer of information between the conscious and the subconscious minds is in how we learn a new skill. When you first learn to drive an automobile, all of your conscious attention is on pressing the gas, steering the car, changing gears, and signalling for turns. In the first months of driving, rolling windows up or down or adjusting a mirror is something attempted only in a parked vehicle. As you gain driving experience, through time the subconscious mind takes over the basic driving functions. One day you find yourself driving with so little conscious thought that you can arrive at your destination and scarcely remember the trip. As your conscious mind was busy thinking of something other than driving, your subconscious mind was controlling the vehicle. Most of the skills that we learn in life, such as writing, reading, typing, bicycling, roller skating, etc., are first learned by the conscious mind, then automatically transferred to the subconscious mind. Automating the use of muscle motor skills is just a small portion of what the subconscious mind is capable of.

The subconscious mind also controls the acid levels in the stomach as well as the assimilation of food into energy. The subconscious mind also regulates the nerve responses and subtle electrical energies in the body.

Although we can attribute many body functions to the subconscious mind, there are many other things that the subconscious mind is capable of that we have not even started to measure. One thing that the subconscious mind does is to regulate the flow and usage of the universal energy around us. It is common knowledge that most of the human race can not enter and actively use their subconscious mind. Once our subconscious mind is linked to the universal energy field around us, healing can be easily initiated. For this to happen, we have to make a link from our conscious mind to the subconscious mind to regulate and control the flow of universal energy.

Metaphysical Secrets for Health and Success in Life

44

Energy all about Us

The Story of Fish

We are creatures that live in a field of energy. We are born in, live, and die within that field of energy, making us totally unaware of the energy field's existence. As a matter of fact, most of the human race denies the existence of the energy field that encompasses the Earth on which we live. But the energy field encompassing the Earth is just a small portion of the expanse of the energy field that fills the entire universe. This energy, which I call 'universal energy' or 'psychic energy', is the matrix which feeds and holds the entire universe together.

Why are we so unaware of the energy field about us? Why do we deny its existence? The reason is that we live within the universal energy field and are totally unaware of energy being around us, just as we are unaware of the air that is around us. If the air about us were removed, we would recognise it missing, as we would suffocate. If we were isolated from the Earth's energy field, we would also experience health effects. A comparable analogy is how fish relate to water. Fish are born, live, and eventually die in water. If you were to ask a fish what water is, the response would be, "What are you talking about?" If you were to try to explain to a fish what water is, it would be hopeless. The average fish that lives in water from life to death has nothing with which to compare its in-the-water existence.

The fish's response would probably be, "We exist like this, we naturally float around as we wish, there is no water around us in our world." If you asked a fish about the surface of the pond, the fish would respond, "That is the end of the world, no one goes there because nothing exists on the other side." Does this sound somehow familiar? From a fish's viewpoint, this is the truth. It is a reality of being a fish. The average fish never leaves the pond. The fish has no other experience to compare to.

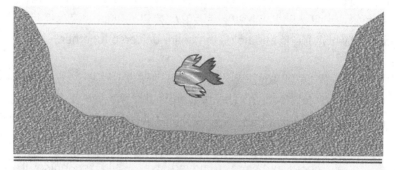

Figure 5.1 The Fish's Known Universe

Let's say one day, as Mr. Fish is swimming along, he grabs onto some food. He instantly finds himself caught on a hook and hauled violently out of the water by a fisherman. Very quickly the fish learns a new reality. It experiences air, the lack of water, and finds that for a fish, this new reality is not a good one. If the fish is lucky enough to escape the hook and return to the water, it now has a new expanded reality that there is more to a fish's life than water. If you grab a hook, you can move out of the reality of water into another reality called air. This fish now has a different experience that proves there is more in life than water. If this fish now tries to share his air experience with his fellow fish, he may find his fellow fish are sceptical and do not believe him. Does this sound familiar to those of you that have had a psychic experience?

The problem of proving the existence of a universal energy in the human existence is very similar to a fish proving to other fish that there is water and air. Very few of us have experienced being separated from the Earth's energy field, either partially or totally. Since we are totally within the universal energy field as a way of existence, we, the fish are likely totally unaware of the energy around us.

How did we become aware of the energy field about us? Where did the concept of universal energy originate? My belief is that the energy levels around the World vary based on geological features present in various areas, the concentration of living entities, and the concentration of non-living entities in the same area.

At some time, individuals sensitive to energy travelled about the Earth and noticed the difference in sensations based on where they were. Further studies over the centuries have revealed more information on the existence of universal energy. Psychic experiences of many different persons around the world have led us to acknowledging the psychic link to universal energy. Psychic energy and universal energy are the same type of energy. The constantly growing base of psychic knowledge had to be dealt with somehow by science. Scientists could not keep ignoring the growing number of psychic experiences involving universal energy or psychic healing. This is probably how the awareness of universal energy came into existence.

You can test this theory by just checking on how you felt in different areas. The feeling of being in a wooded area with many living trees and plants about can be very energizing. The plants emit large amounts of universal energy that can easily be assimilated into living bodies. This is why practitioners of stress management always suggest a walk in the woods to calm jagged nerves. The foliage always does the job of relaxing and transmitting healing energy to us.

The feeling in a shopping mall can be very tiring and draining. This is because an enclosed shopping mall is devoid of adequate foliage to balance the lack of energy in the surroundings from the human-made structure and artificial ventilation. Also, the shopping mall's energy field contains erratic energy transmitted by the people in the shopping mall while they are in the midst of a shopping frenzy. The resulting mall atmosphere is a very personally draining one as compared to the calm, serene forest setting. The degree and quality of the universal energy are very quickly felt when going from a forest area directly to a shopping mall. Our personal feelings are directly affected based on that same degree and quality of universal energy about us. Check the theory for yourself. Are there places that feel bad, resulting in your just not wanting to be there? This is due to an absence of psychic energy at that location. Are there places that feel good and you tend to spend as much time there as you can? It could be because of how you interact with the quality and your compatibility with the universal energy in that location.

If you fly long distances, you can suffer from jet lag. Jet lag is caused by your body adjusting to the different universal energy configurations between the two locations. A plane moves people physically too quickly between the two areas for the passengers' bodies to adjust to the subtle changes of universal energy about them. This is the phenomenon that we call jet lag. Prior to high-speed travel, people walked or rode horses. Their bodies had ample time to adjust to the energy changes about them, as the changes were more gradual. Travel fatigue started with trains and automobiles. We thought the shaking around within the vehicle was the main cause of travel fatigue. I would like to suggest that in fact travel fatigue is also a by-product of our body's inability to cope with the rapid energy changes we experience while travelling.

Although we all experience feeling universal energy, many of us are unaware of it. We can feel the energy about us, but science tells us that it cannot be measured, so it may just not be there. There is still a problem with scientifically proving the existence of universal psychic energy. Even our latest technology cannot measure quantitatively psychic energy or universal energy.

The Fish in an Electric Sea

Are we just like fish living in an electric sea? Can psychic energy be electrical energy, or is electrical energy a crude component of psychic energy? Everyone has experienced the effect of what is called static electricity one time or another in their life. The simple explanation for static electricity is that it is caused by the friction between two dissimilar materials that results in an electrical discharge. This simple explanation leads to a larger question. Is lightning static electricity caused by two clouds rubbing together in the same way as wool rubbing against nylon causes a spark? The answer is both yes and no.

Above the Earth at about 60 miles is the Ionosphere. Between the Ionosphere and the Earth is the air that we breathe. Air is electrically semi-conductive depending on the level of electricity and the humidity of the air. You measure the potential difference across the two ends of a battery and get a power reading. This same concept can be applied to the surface of the Earth and the Ionosphere 60 miles up. The electrical difference between the Earth's surface and the Ionosphere has been estlmated to be about 400,000 volts at a rating of 1,800 amperes. The air in between that we breathe is an insulator that keeps the two charges separated. It has been said that our 60-mile high atmosphere acts as an electrical insulator with the insulation value or electrical resistance of 200 ohms. If the air about us has an insulation value of about 200 ohms, it is slowing down the movement of electrical energy flow from the Ionosphere to the Earth but not stopping it, as 200 ohms is a relatively low resistance factor.

In electrical theory fundamentals, the Earth is always considered the ground or the negative side of the battery. The way that we control an out-of-control electrical charge is to ground it, which simply means stick the hot end of the wire into the Earth or, in electrical terms, to the ground. This would tend to lead us to believe that the air around us is positively charged and the Earth we live on is negatively charged. If this is so, then we are really like fish living in an ocean of positive electrical charges. The air around us that we breathe can be an actual ocean of electrical energy. I personally believe that electrical energy is just a component of the universal or psychic energy that surrounds us. We go about our daily lives usually totally unaware of the subtle energy that surrounds us. If the rotation of the Earth dragging against the atmosphere results in friction, causing the Ionosphere to have a positively charged atmosphere, where does it leave us in the electrical realm of things?

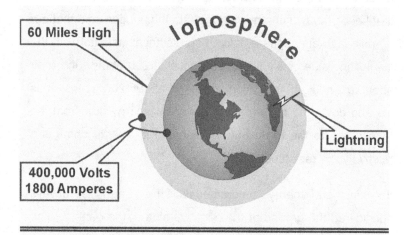

Figure 5.2 Earth's Electrical Field

Since we are grounded by the simple contact with the Earth, we probably take on the charge of the Earth, which is a negative charge. This is an important theory because it best explains the auras that some people see and most people can sense. If we are in contact with the Earth, the Earth's energy field will be modified in the area immediately around us. It is most likely that the negative charge that covers the Earth's surface also connects with bodies. Because of humankind's sense of this phenomenon, some unique statements have come forward, such as Mother Earth, grounding yourself, hug a tree, etc. The list goes on and on, but the basic concept is that we as a race have sensed the subtle energy fields around us and have developed axioms from intuitive knowledge to help ourselves subconsciously use the surrounding energy without consciously having to foster any belief in the energy field.

The Charge of Vitality

Before we continue talking about the electrical ionization of the atmosphere, there is one thing that should be first clarified. A negative ion charge is an electronic and physics term that is not related to positive and negative energy as stated in psychic terms. The technical term is based on electrical polarity theory and is just a scientific value that was chosen as a scientific value.

In the psychic field, we have chosen to use the terms positive and negative feeling as a way to describe how we affect or are affected by others. Feelings, whether positive or negative, from another individual are encoded messages that we perceive. These encoded feeling messages may be transferred in the form of an electrical charge, whether the charge stated in technical terms is positive or negative. In this book we are stating the positive or negative charge as in technical terminology and not as related to feelings. To simplify the matter when dealing with feelings, we will use different terminology.

There have been studies on the effects of electrical ionization, which, simply put, is the study of how the human body reacts to the electrical charges about us. Around us the atmosphere is composed of a subtle charge of positive electrical ions which we interact with all the time. It is the thin negative ion charge that coats our body from contact with the Earth that allows us to effectively deal with these natural charges.

Known Benefits of Negative Ions

- *Increase personal performance, improve work capacity.*

- *Give a cheerful disposition, increase a person's reaction time.*

- *Aid in relieving or reducing the effects of allergies.*

- *Enhance metabolism.*

- *Relieve pain.*

- *Aid in healing.*

- *Aid in personal physical balance.*

- *Aid in speeding up burn treatment.*

However, the invention of electrical appliances and machines has changed the amount of positive ions that we interact with each and every day. Most electrical devices create a positive charge of ions around them as they operate. All the electrical devices that are around you at home, at work, or at play probably encompass you in an atmosphere that is extremely charged with positive ions. There have been studies noting the health effects of ions on the human body, and the effects of positive ions are not encouraging. Living in a rich positive ion atmosphere can result in decreased personal performance, depression, loss of intuition, and increased length of personal reaction time. This may be the reason why people who live in urban centres and cities suffer far more from depression and emotional burnout. These medical problems may not be caused by a hectic lifestyle; they may just be a result of living in a high electrically positive charged environment.

Negative ions have also been studied and the results have found them to be more helpful than positive ions.

It almost sounds like exposure to negative ions is the miracle cure. Living in nature's atmosphere of negative ions is really not a miracle cure but the normal lifestyle that our mechanized society has abandoned.

As we are all committed to a lifestyle based on our personal circumstances, it may just not be practical to pack up and drop all your commitments to live the lifestyle of a priest or Eastern monk, unfettered by the energies of modern society. There are some things that we can do to achieve a more balanced lifestyle. The first thing is to be aware of and manage the electrical ions about us to create a more habitable environment around us.

If negative ions are so important to our survival, where do we find them? How do we use them? Using negative ions is the easy part. All that we have to do is be in the physical location of negative ions to reap the benefits of their effect. Seems simple enough, but where do we find these ions?

In a forest or near trees and plants is an excellent source of negative ions. Plants generate negative ions as well as being producers of oxygen and absorbers of carbon dioxide. Spend some time in parks or in the country. You will quickly feel the life-enhancing effects. You may wish to bring the forest home in the form of houseplants. This will change the ion charges in your living space. By standing in the area of influence of an object that generates negative ions, you can enhance your general health and mental state. Just by standing or sitting under a tree you can absorb the energy field and enhance your state of being. Waterfalls are an excellent source of negative ions. Actually, any form of flowing water can produce negative ions. Spend some time sitting by a waterfall or a natural stream in the country and you will feel the relaxing effect that it can have on you. Many people install fountains in their homes to create water flow that creates negative ions. It is most likely that even with the use of a fountain's low-power positive ion producing electrical pump, a fountain's water flow is capable of producing more negative ions than positive ions.

Other forms of negative ion generators may be ponds or fish tanks where there is a flow of water. It has been known that people have found sitting by a pond or looking into a fish tank to be very relaxing.

Burning a candle can create negative ions. An age-old axiom is to burn a candle to remove any bad influences in a person's life. I would like to suggest that candle burning is more practical than mystical. If burning a candle creates negative ions, it will make the atmosphere more relaxing, thus aid, in the removing of bad feelings or depression. If a person is more relaxed, it has been found that their natural psychic abilities become enhanced. This simple fact may be the basis for the use of candles in many rituals and ceremonies.

If the natural methods of creating a negative ion atmosphere about you are not practical for your lifestyle, you may consider purchasing an electrical negative ion generator. This apparatus will create a negative ion atmosphere that will benefit your health, but be aware that, although this machine can enhance your atmosphere, it is still an electrical machine and does affect your environment as any electrical machine would.

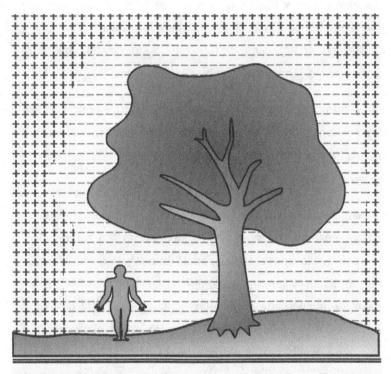

Figure 5.3 Natural Negative Ion Charge from Trees

Another method of enhancing your living space is to minimize the use of electrical appliances that create positive ions. If a radio or television is not in use for long periods of time, unplug it. Although the unit may not be used, the transformer in it may still be circulating electricity. If you use two refrigerators for convenience, conserve by using one. Reduce use of air conditioning on the days that an open window can be used to circulate and cool the air in your home. Many of the things that you can do to limit your exposure to electricity can also enhance your lifestyle. So make your environment healthier and save a few dollars along the way.

Kirlian Photography

Currently, the only repeatable method of scientifically measuring psychic energy is through the use of Kirlian photography. Kirlian photography has been used for a number of years to take energy pictures. The scientific community still debates what Kirlian photography pictures are. Some say it is a picture of heat emanations, some say it is an electrical charge based on the Kirlian photography process, and still say that the picture is a residual electrical imprint. The scientific use of Kirlian photography is still debated. The fact still holds that Kirlian photography gives repeatable physical results of something that relates to an undefined energy that we currently cannot scientifically explain.

One of the problems that we live with is that even though our civilization is very technically advanced, some technologies are still very crude. We still have no way to measure a feeling, a thought, or an idea. Anything dealing with human senses is difficult to quantify and accurately measure. Human senses are still the only way to detect and measure subtle psychic energy. Our present mechanical and electrical measuring devices cannot measure psychic energy with any repeatable results, if they can measure psychic energy at all. The crudeness of this equipment causes us not to be able to measure what is there and unseen by most people. The scientific community will not accept something that cannot be repeatedly demonstrated, mechanically measured, and explained to the finest detail. As a result, universal psychic energy is recognised as an unproven fact or non-fact. Even though universal psychic energy is used on a regular basis for healing, it could not be scientifically proven; therefore it does not scientifically exist.

Building Blocks of the Universe

Atomic Structure

Since the atom was split, we have moved into a new age of knowledge. The atom, which was known as that microscopic piece that everything of the universe is made of, could be located and split apart. Interestingly enough, the reaction from destroying such a minute particle was enormous. The enormous energy released by splitting the atom was demonstrated when the first atomic bomb was dropped. The results were devastating. Humankind currently employs and continues to research the use of atomic energy. We consistently split atoms to create large discharges of energy to create heat for operating electrical turbine generators, for large ship and submarine propulsion, to name just a few uses.

Although the splitting of atoms gives us energy, what is the real cost? We are systematically breaking small bits of the universe up without knowing what the long-term effect may be. The toxic residue from splitting atoms has severe radiation effects on all types of matter, with a long period of poisonous activity attached to it. Atomic fusion appears to be an up-to-date power source as well as having an unknown effect on the universe's energy field we live in. No one today knows the long-term result of splitting atoms, in the same way as the pioneers of the combustion engine did not know that the long-term result of their invention would be to poison the air we breathe and that their invention would eventually be a major contributor to the greenhouse effect on the Earth of today.

To minimize the destructive use of the Earth's energy field, we need to use less electricity. Although we greatly depend on electricity, it is still debatable whether it is safe to use. In recent years we have had the technology to study the subtle effects of magnetic fields on the human body. Through various studies, it has been found that the magnetic pulses from electrical motors as small as ceiling fans could inflict long-term health effects upon us.

The electricity model is probably one of the best to use for illustration, as it so very closely parallels the use of the psychic energy in the universe about us. The way that we can make electricity flow with mechanical devices is paralleled with how our bodies can generate and produce psychic energy in the universe.

Nothing Lost, Nothing Gained

One basic law in the universe is that energy cannot be created or lost. Even in the case of atomic energy, the great release of energy from atom splitting is a matter of changing the form of an atom, which results in a large release of energy. What other repercussions the dissemination of the atom has we cannot measure to date. As we carry on further in our study, keep this important point in mind: that energy can not be created out of nothing. Energy comes from somewhere and eventually will go somewhere. When an atom is split, a magnetic pulse is discharged which does destroy matter and perhaps a section of the matrix that the universe is created from.

When we look at the electron theory of how a charge on something such as a battery can move electrons in a subtle manner through a wire so that electricity is formed, we can see how a transfer of energy collected by the movements of electrons can be achieved. With our ever-growing technology, it has been found that electric motors and some common electrical appliances can emit an electrical pulse that can create a poor effect on a person's health. Just imagine the residual effect of an atomic device when billions of electrons are violently surged through the magnetic pulse. As fish in an electric sea, we are affected by any energy disruption which ripples out through that electric sea. The effectual physical distance and long-term effects of our atomic and electric devices are still not really known.

As the fish lives in water and is totally unaware of the water, it can be unknowingly poisoned through a slow introduction of pollutants. We, as humans in a physical world, can suffer the same poisoning from the slow changing of our energy environment, without our actually sensing the change. Although our bodies are designed to adapt, there is a limit to the adaptive process, where disease and sickness start to become the norm. As humans living in the electric sea, we must raise our awareness of our interaction with electrical devices and learn to manage these same electrical appliances.

What can we do to minimize the effect of mechanical and electrical energy influences on our life? The best way is to live away from a city, as in a rural setting there are fewer electrical lines and devices to affect you. This is why Eastern religious teachers live in remote areas of India and Tibet, totally unhampered by the energies of city life. If moving to a rural community is not realistic for you, the next best thing to do is to spend as much time as you can in a park or in the woods. Take some time each day to be there quietly to re-energize your body from the energies from the grass, flowers and trees.

Optimizing Your Energy Environment

We all live with appliances as a part of our industrialized lifestyle. Minimize the use of electrical appliances that you depend upon. When any electrical device is not in use, unplug it. Most electrical devices such as televisions, radios, etc. have transformers in them that operate even when the device is turned off. So if you are not using an electrical appliance, unplug it to remove an unneeded electro-magnetic field in your living space. You will make your living space environmentally friendlier and save a little hydro money as well.

Our civilization is so dependent on electrical devices that it may not be possible to change the tide of public opinion about whether we should use electrical power as an energy source or investigate other sources of power. The good news is that our current technology has made great bounds in identifying and putting into place many revolutionary changes that will effectively reduce the amount of electricity used to power our electrical toys. Many products boast low power usage, low ionization output, low radiation output, etc., etc. With each new generation of electrical devices, inventors find ways to make them more efficient, safer, and more environmentally friendly. The bonus derived from these new products is a continually lower consumption of electrical power. The downside of this efficiency is that more and more people are using electrical devices, so that the designed energy savings are balanced out by the wider spread use of electrical products. Because more people are using electrical products, it is more important today than ever to manage your personal exposure to the appliances that you use and own.

Are Auras Real or Fiction?

Throughout history, psychics and seers have proclaimed to see auras or feel energies from living things. Through the ages, these sensitive people have observed things that the masses have either not noticed or learned to ignore. The scientific community has at times also captured glimpses of the energy which we call auras.

Our physical bodies are usually considered to be just a collection of tissue types. Humankind is usually referred to as skin and bone. The interesting part of our make-up is that our bodies are also comprised of various minerals. Two of these minerals are iron and salt. It has been found that a lack of iron or salt in a person's physical make-up can cause tremendous physical disorders and, in severe cases, death. As our bodies are composed of these elements that can create and conduct energy, it only follows that that we must carry a personal energy field. The following topics will explore various theories of energy transfer that apply to our physical condition.

Humankind as Magnets

If we look more closely at the elements in our bodies, we find that the iron component is a conductor of electricity and magnetism. Could it be that the lack of iron in our bodies stops the life-giving flow of the energy around us? Could the flow of this energy through us be as important to our survival as food? We know that the Earth has magnetic properties and lines of natural magnetism. The metals in our bodies surely respond to

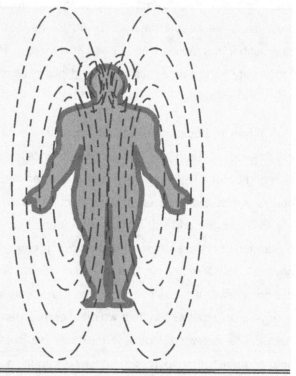

Figure 7.1 The Body's Magnetic Field Described by Early Chinese Medicine.

this magnetic influence, as we have an iron content in our bodies. The electromagnetic devices that we choose to surround ourselves with can also have an influence on our body's magnetic content. There is a healing treatment where people wear high-intensity magnets. The magnetic fields from these magnets act as a health aid to reduce pain and as a result elevate the general level of physical well-being. Magnetic therapy is a field that fills many volumes of information if you wish to pursue that avenue of study. It is interesting that a consistent magnetic field is said to be health enhancing but magnetism created by flowing electricity is considered harmful to our health.

Humankind as Crystals

Another vital element of life is salt. Salt in its natural state is a crystal. Crystals have been used in crystal radios to receive radio transmissions. People, under certain conditions, have also been able to hear radio transmissions without the aid of any radio equipment. Crystals have been used to convert physical energy into electrical energy. Ruby crystals are used in lasers to direct the energy of the laser beam. Silicon is another crystal that is used in computers and electronics. People have also been known to generate electrical charges. There are many volumes written on the metaphysical uses of crystals as well as the health benefits related to the wearing of crystals. Crystals influence the subtler realm of human energy in a much similar fashion as they do in radio transmitters. It is no wonder that crystals have been used for centuries to foretell events, aid in healing, as well as being instruments of the metaphysical arts.

Any attribute that can be given to a crystal is also inherent in our physical bodies, as we contain salt and other mineral crystals in our bloodstream. Those subtle energies that affect crystals, such as various kinds of radio waves and electronic pulses, can also affect our physical bodies.

Humankind as Water

Our bodies are comprised of a high percentage of water. Water is an element that makes life possible on this planet. Any living thing that exists on this planet is more than likely to have a water component in its make-up. Since water is an excellent conductor of electrical energy, it follows that electrical energy about us can influence our health and well-being.

What Does It All Mean?

The list of uses for the mineral crystals and water present in our bodies is quite extensive. The point is that the elements that our bodies are comprised of are quite extensive. These very same elements are known to be quite capable of harnessing, storing, and using electrical, magnetic, and any other energy that is available for use. As the fish in the electric sea, we are so accustomed to and interconnected with the energy fields around us that we simply do not pay any attention to them.

The only danger in using manufactured energy is that we have not explored the effects on the body's natural energy field. We do not know to what extent the human body is affected by human-made energy sources. We do know that the body can readily absorb nuclear energy to the point of our demise, but there is no danger associated with absorbing the nature's energies as transmitted by forestry, common crystals, and plants. Since humankind has done damage to our Ionosphere, absorption of the sun's life-giving energy must be done in moderation. The heat generated by the sun is essential to existence of humankind. Age-old sun treatment has been used in the past for enhancing health, but now, with the degeneration of the ozone layer, exposure to the sun has changed from a healthy method of energy gathering to exposing oneself to an energy source that must be respected and used with intentionally and sparingly.

Our Immediate Energy Field

About us is the electric sea of energy, and, having life, we also generate internal energy. Each of us has a unique energy field from the interaction of our personal internal energy and the atmospheric energy about us. This unique energy field has been considered as body heat, personal space, as well as various types of energy. This energy field is similar to that shown in Figure7.2. This energy profile actually leads us to the belief that a human energy field, called an aura, can actually exist.

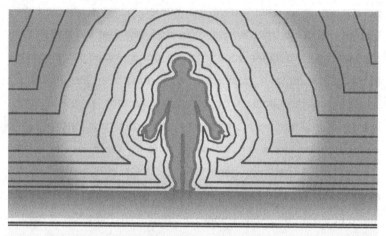

Figure 7.2 The Unseen Power of the Unconscious Mind

Auras and Energy Fields

If there is energy all about us, then there must be a way to use our body to harness and control that energy. Many people have stated that they have seen auras. An aura is what is considered a psychic energy field generated by a person's body. For centuries psychics have talked of auras and claimed to have seen or sensed energy fields about other people's bodies. Most of the world's population have not made such claims or believe in a human body energy field. I would like to propose that it is not only possible but also highly probable that people have energy fields around them that they actually can control. If the air about us is charged with positive ions and the Earth has a negative ion charge, our bodies are then the intermediate conductors of energy between the Earth and the air. By manipulating the elements in our physical bodies we can use the surrounding energies in some unique ways that we cannot duplicate or measure with machines.

Nikola Tesla

In energy research, first Carlson, then Nikola Tesla discovered that there is a subtle energy that is present in the human body. It was claimed that Nikola Tesla had such understanding of the human body that he could actually conduct vast amounts of electrical energy through his body. Nikola Tesla, in his scientific pursuit, may have touched upon discovering some of the same energy centres that Eastern philosophy has recognized for centuries. Nikola Tesla mapped three major energy centres within the human body that he believed were electrical centres of the body. Since the work of Nikola Tesla, many other scientists and medical professionals have worked with the electrical elements within the human body. Indeed electricity is present and flows through our bodies.

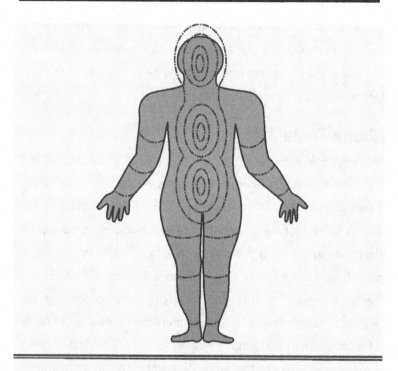

Figure 7.3 The Body's Energy Field as Described by Carlson and Tesla

Chakras

Over the centuries, Eastern disciplines have recognized the energy centres within our bodies by the name of Chakra. The human body has numerous energy centres throughout it, but there are six commonly recognized major energy centres. These centres are believed to control different aspects of our physical, emotional, and spiritual being. These major energy centres are in positions of relatively the same locations as major organs. The brow, heart, and spleen Chakras appear to be in the same body locales as the three major energy centres discovered by Tesla and Carlson. There are many other interpretations of the number of major Chakras in the human body. This is because the human body has over two hundred energy centres. People have been known to develop other of these energy centres into the size of a major Chakra due to life events. This would be why the various writings differ on the number of Chakras and Chakra locations.

If Chakras are the energy centres of the body, a whole new dimension on how we view health and life must be addressed. We know that if our bodies cool down enough we will freeze and our bodies will shut down. Until now, the element of physical heat has been measured as a temperature source. Our temperature is one of the first things that a medical doctor checks to measure our level of health. I would like to propose that the energy level vital to health is not measured only in degrees of temperature but also in the amount of universal psychic energy that the body's Chakra points contain. We operate our bodies by electrical impulses running through our nervous system. If our reserve of Chakra energy is low, the supply of energy to operate our body's nervous system will be low. This state of low energy can lead to illness and the emergence of real physical medical conditions.

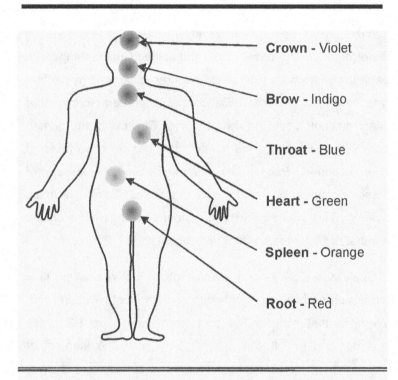

Figure 7.4 The Chakra Energy Centers as Described by Eastern Philosophy

One way of preserving a high level of health is to maintain a balanced Chakra system of energy. Balanced Chakra energy not only balances the physical body but also maintains a stable emotional level of being. If you wish to have and maintain good health and a general feeling of well-being, the method to achieve this is by balancing the Chakra energy centres. Heat and temperature are by-products of application of energy. When we measure a person's temperature, are we in fact measuring health by the by-product of health and not recognizing the real element of life, the internal Chakra energy? Many spiritual practitioners hold to the premise, that if you heal the body's chakra energy centres, good physical health will follow. Can it be that we are medically treating physical symptoms for good health and not following the actual source of good health? I do not suggest that we should abandon medical assistance when necessary, but rather that we should use energy management as a method of enhancing medical treatment. The best use of energy management is as a preventative health measure.

Balancing the Chakras

To balance our Chakras, we have to look back at the iceberg model to gain clues on how to influence our personal energy centres. The body's Chakras are regulated by the hidden part of the iceberg called the subconscious mind. Our subconscious thought patterns and the Chakra energy settings recorded in our personal universal maps regulate energy or lack of energy in the Chakra energy centres. To gain access to regulation of the system of Chakras within our bodies, we need to create a bridge from the conscious mind to the subconscious mind. The most effective method of balancing Chakras is through the use of meditation. Meditation is simply assuming a restful position in a quiet place and directing your thoughts to a specific purpose. In this case, the purpose would be to balance your

Chakra system. The tool used during meditation is our imagination. Imagination is the unseen link between our conscious and subconscious minds.

The proceeding is a simple Chakra Meditation that can be employed for Chakra balancing. It works well if you record it on a personal recorder in a soft voice at a slow pace. Then play it back during your meditation session. You could also have someone else read the meditation for you, but you will find it more effective if it is heard in your voice, as your subconscious mind follows directions more readily from within than from other people. With some practice you can use this meditation from memory with the same type of results. To do the meditation, find a comfortable location. It should be a quiet place where you can relax and not be disturbed. Preferably the location will be free of electronic appliances and telephones that can ring. To set the tone for a peaceful mood, have the area lit dimly and take a relaxing position by sitting in a soft chair or, if you choose lie down on a comfortable surface.

The Chakra Meditation

Close your eyes and relax. If you have any stiff muscles, give them a light stretch to relax them. Once you are relaxed, with your eyes closed, imagine in your mind's eye that you see your body. As you see your body in your imagination you notice some balls of light that are different colours that appear to be in a series from the top of your head to the base of your spine. As you observe these energy centres in your body, you realise that they are the Chakra Centres which regulate your health. As you look at these centres you may observe one or more of them that are not as bright or strong as the others are. If you notice this, it is time to adjust the weaker energy centre(s) up to the brightness of the others. To do this, imagine that you have found a control knob for the weak Chakra (energy centre). Turn the knob clockwise until the weak centre becomes as brilliant as the rest of the energy centres. Repeat this procedure until all of the Chakra Energy Centres are of an equal brilliance.

(PAUSE)

The Chakra Meditation (continued)

Remember to always adjust your Chakras to increase the brilliance of light to increase your physical and emotional health. Once all of your energy centres are balanced, take some time to relax and enjoy the feeling of being balanced.

(PAUSE)

When you are ready, slowly move your arms and legs and then open your eyes.

Note: As you are working with your imagination with your conscious mind linked to your subconscious mind, it may take a few moments to leave the relaxed state. All people use their imagination in different ways. You may see the energy centres in your mind's eye as you adjust them in your imagination. Alternately, you may not see the energy centres in your imagination but are able to feel the centres and adjust them based on your feelings or sensations. The way your imagination operates is based on your personal map. If you wish to use your imagination in a different manner, it is time to review your personal universal map and revise how you want your imagination to operate.

The Chakra Meditation is not a once-in-a-lifetime adjustment. As we go through life and face many challenges, we regularly need to adjust our Chakras to resist the pressures and influences of our surrounding environment. By using the Chakra Meditation on a regular basis, you will find that your life will run better.

How Big is Our Personal Energy Field?

Our Chakras and nervous systems generate energy, but as the fish in the electric sea, it does not stop within our body. The energy in our bodies contacts and intermingles with the energy of the Earth and the atmosphere. The area where intermingling of energy occurs can be described as the aura. Every living thing has an aura. Our body's aura operates the same way as the Chakras as an indicator of an individual's health. The energy mixing about our bodies breaks personal auras into three levels. These three aura levels relate to health and mental well-being. All people can sense the effect of the aura. How you sense an aura depends on how you view psychic energy based on your personal universal map.

Whether we like it or not, the energy field that is around us, is a component of health and how we relate to other people. The aura is what a psychic uses to sense the untold and invisible facets of our personal being. The aura about us is an energy field which is as real as an electrical charge or the pull of a magnet.   In the same way a magnetometer measures a magnetic field, a psychic senses and reads an Aura.

The Structure of the Aura

The aura is broken into three levels. Each level has a different intensity and reflects on different aspects of your physical and emotional being. It is said that all that affects us, past, present, future, health, mental well-being, illness, etc., can be sensed within our aura. As we are the fish that live in the electric sea, it makes sense that our personal energy field should appear in the electric sea in the form of an aura. The aura's three distinct

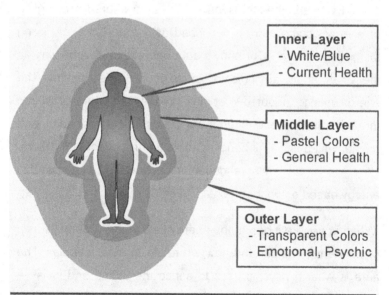

Inner Layer
- White/Blue
- Current Health

Middle Layer
- Pastel Colors
- General Health

Outer Layer
- Transparent Colors
- Emotional, Psychic

Figure 7.5 The Aura as Described by Eastern Philosophy

layers are formed from the energy blend of the two energy fields. Each of these three layers contains different things about your being that can be sensed by a psychic or intuitively sensitive individual.

Inner Aura Layer

The layer of your Aura that is in contact with your body is the strongest, and the most intense as it is the one that conducts the energy of your body. This layer is also fortified by our body's contact with the Earth. The ion energy that flows from the air about us into the Earth is the most intense around our body, as this is where the mainstream of energy flow occurs. The consistency of this layer is a measurement of your current emotional/physical energy level. The stronger this layer of energy is, the better your current general health is. If a person is currently physically ill, this inner aura layer is the one that psychic healing practitioners sense as weak and work to fortify with additional psychic or universal energy. The strength of this inner aura layer is also a measure of your body's ability to resist physical and mental illness. By monitoring and building up this aura layer, you will protect yourself from illness and mental depression. The inner layer of your aura is the layer that when sensed by others, will depict your present health and life force. Most psychic healing techniques employ revitalising or building up of the universal energy charge on this inner aura layer.

Middle Aura Layer

The middle aura layer consists of a transparent pastel colouring. Most people who have been trained can usually sense this layer of the aura. This is the section of your aura that signifies what your general health conditions are. By interpreting this aura layer, natural healers can sense your current health condition. Also, observing inconsistencies in the aura can show what can be brewing up for your health in the future. Inconsistencies in the aura are actually energy indicators of where a disease will likely manifest itself. An interesting thought is whether disease is first transferred from person to person in the form of energy which can manifest itself in mental or physical illness on a future date. Another theory is that disease finds its way through a hole in the aura. If a psychic can sense an upcoming illness from your aura, then it follows that a weak aura is a weak personal energy field that may lead to the physical acceptance of an illness or virus.

Outer Aura Layer

The outer aura layer is the part of your personal energy field with which you psychically and emotionally interact with the world on an energy basis. This part of your aura is your invisible psychic antenna that senses the sublime invisible energy world of premonition and the sixth sense. From time to time everyone has had a feeling or a notion of something and later you found, the event actually happened at a later date. This occurs because the outer aura layer connects with either another aura or energy field containing that particular information. That connection transfers thoughts or images into your subconscious mind. By extending the outer aura field, we can visualize things at a distance, pick up electronic transmissions, or sense others' thoughts and motives.

When a person enters your personal space, this aura layer is what they are entering. That is why it is so important to avoid being in the proximity of people that have bad mental dispositions, as their aura energy can be mixed with yours. The saying, 'What has rubbed off on you' may be more fact than jest in the use of psychic energy.

Auras and the Electron Theory

The electron theory based on the atomic structure of all things is a model of the microscopic universe. I like to refer to this initial point to understand how the psychic energy field about us operates and how we as individuals and groups in this physical world can influence this field.

The electron theory works on the simple premise that each atom is composed of small particles called electrons, which rotate about a core called the nucleus. The electrons can be kicked out of their orbit and moved when an external force is exerted on them. The force to move electrons can be induced by the use of a chemical reaction, as in a battery, or by a physical mechanical energy, such as is exerted on a generator. Once these electrons are flowing, it is said that we have electricity.

As the atoms are the building blocks of the universe, all matter is composed of atoms as a common element. This means that if we can mentally induce thoughts to affect the electrons in ourselves or any other element in the universe, we can then mentally influence how the physical world and events around us are shaped. This powerful idea means that the very thought any of us has in our head at this moment can be rippling out through the universe, as rings on the surface of a pond caused by dropping in a pebble. These rings make an ever-expanding circular ripple in the water that will grow until eventually passes over the whole pond, touching the entire shoreline. Using the electron theory, it is possible to surmise that thoughts can be generated with the same energy ripple effect. This means that psychic impressions of the future can come from the ripples of energy that people expel today.

We live in the physical world, but the real connections that we have are on the atomic electron energy level. Through this energy we are connected to everyone and everything in the entire universe.

Just imagine all the people that you are in contact with every day share the same energy field that you do. If they are carrying energy of ill intent with them, your contact with them will pick up some of that energy, and it will automatically blend with yours. The result will be that you can carry around a bad feeling or attitude that you have received from another individual that you interacted with. This natural energy mix is shown in Figure 7.6

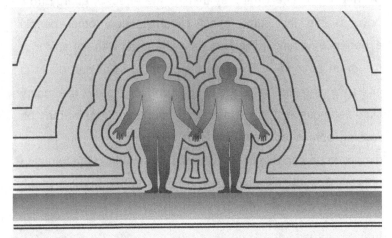

Figure 7.6 The Unseen Effect of Shared Unseen Energy

How does this compare with our personal aura? If we live in an electric sea, then it follows that our personal aura is an electric field generated or controlled by our physical body. With this in mind, it is possible to use our bodies to control our auras as a psychic tool to direct and use psychic energy as easily as a kitchen appliance uses electricity to cook food. If the electron theory holds true, then it follows that our bodies simply control electrons to create and manage our auras.

Auras and Spirits

A spirit has no aura because it has no way of controlling the electron energy field in which we live. This is a really important point to remember in the case of haunting. In a haunting, some people experience what they think is the effect of energy from beyond. In the same exact circumstances, other people experience nothing. This has very little to do with the spirits or the great beyond. The only thing that a spirit can do is to influence the thoughts of a person to create the scary circumstances that are related to a haunting. A spirit may be wishing only to communicate with a living person, but fear in that living person of what they sense can manifest the haunting effect. A spirit has absolutely no power in the physical world, except that which we give it.

Persons who are afflicted with mental disease or are plagued with spirits may only be persons that cannot control their personal energy field and leave it as a playground for discarnate entities to use or abuse.

Mediums well understand that a spirit cannot affect them. Mediums are trained in personal energy management, which allows them to tune their auras so they can receive accurate messages from spirits. When done properly, there are no effects of the spirits controlling physical surroundings with the medium's personal energy. Any physical effects and noises are usually caused by the observer's lack of energy control. The medium, in fact, can take control of the observer's energy to stop the spirit effect and noises.

Aura Cleansing

Your aura is your personal energy field that you must take control of if you wish to achieve peace, harmony, or success in this life. As we go through life, we pick up things in our Aura from physical surroundings and other people. If you are around happy people, you leave with a good feeling and part of their joy. If you are around sad people, you pick up a bit of their pain and misery. Just by being alive and interacting with the world we pickup all kinds of energy. Although energy transfer happens, there is no reason to carry the bad thought or bad feeling energy around with us. We can at any time take a few minutes and psychically wash out the bad energy from our aura by using the following simple, but effective, technique to clean our Aura.

The following meditation can be done at any time you feel tense, tired, ill, or in a bad mood. All you need is a few minutes in a quiet place to cleanse your aura by this method to revitalize yourself.

Aura Cleansing Technique

Sit quietly in a chair with your eyes closed and visualize in your mind's eye, that you are in a shower of white light coming down from the sky above you, that is washing you clean like a shower. As the white light showers you, notice how the air around you (your aura if you can sense it) gets cleaned as well. Feel the air (aura) around you get lighter and clearer. Let the energy shower flow relaxed energy into your physical body and relax. Do this until you relax and feel yourself breathing with little effort. Then slowly wake yourself with three deep breaths and then move as you feel comfortable to do.

Energy Management

Energy Input

Our personal energy comes from a number of elements. To exist in this physical world we require external energy input. This input is broken into basically three energy sources: air, food, and universal energy. With a balance of our external energy input, we can live a healthy life. Deprivation or over-indulgence of these elements can lead to health problems and, in some cases, death. The energy inputs are required for life and are also required for the ability to do the things that we wish to achieve in this life.

Air

The most basic source of energy is the air about us. Without the air, we would lack oxygen and, as a result, could not survive. Yoga masters of the East believe that other than oxygen, the air we breathe contains a subtle energy called prana. To extract this prana from the air about us, we can use the same breathing exercises used by the mystics. Prana can be used to re-energize your body, collect additional personal energy, and use universal psychic energy for healing. The following exercise can be used to extract pranic energy from the air about us. This exercise can be done standing or sitting, with your eyes open or shut. It can be done quickly and easily anywhere.

91

With practice of this technique, you can build up the duration time of the segments from three seconds to five seconds and the number of repetitions from three to five.

Prana Exercise

Sit or stand quietly with your eyes closed. Take a deep breath. Inhale for 3 seconds. Hold the air in your lungs for 3 seconds. Exhale for 3 seconds. Pause for 3 seconds, then inhale for 3 seconds. Repeat this cycle 3 times.

Food

The next basic survival item is food. Without air, we would cease to exist in a matter of minutes. Without food, we would cease to exist in a matter of days. The nutrients that we survive on are extracted by our bodies from the food that we eat and the water we drink. Besides the chemical attributes that are in the foods we eat, there is also an energy component that our body consumes. The quality of the food we eat needs to be measured for nutrients and universal psychic energy to get the best total nourishment for our physical well-being.

One of the prime considerations in gaining universal psychic energy from food is that the lower the processing of the food item, the higher the living energy component. If you wish to have better health and a higher energy level, pursue a high vegetable diet. Raw vegetables and fruit are the best sources of living energy that can be eaten.

Another method of energizing your food is to bless it before eating. Blessing your food before eating it can attune it to your body so that you can get the best value out of the food. Blessing food can also remove any bad feelings that may be present from contact the food had with the person who prepared it. Since everything we eat has been alive, or should have been, a blessing is vital to expressing thanks for the sacrifice of the living entity so that we can physically survive. Blessings are to be said respectfully, with your eyes closed in front of the food. The following are a couple of simple blessings that you can use. Use the one of your preference, or make up a personalized one for yourself.

Food Blessing 1

'Lord, thank you for this food and please bless it for our personal use.'

Food Blessing 2

May the Universal Source cleanse this food for my personal use.

Universal Energy

We live in a field of energy. Whether we consciously draw upon universal energy or not, we still use it. It is a known fact that space travel out of the Earth's energy field results in a number of health effects. I would like to suggest that coexistence with the Earth's energy field is a natural symbiotic relationship which is vital to our physical existence. The various energy elements have been discussed in earlier chapters. We draw in and use universal psychic energy as a component that is vital to our existence. Some techniques of gathering and using this energy will be covered in subsequent chapters. All that is required to know at this point is that we take in, use, and expel psychic energy in the same way as we do any other energy.

Sunlight is another energy that is vital to our existence. We gather light energy as well as some vitamins from the sun, but in recent years, with the thinning of the atmosphere, overexposure to the sun can have a toxic effect. Absorption of sunlight has to be done with careful measure. An actual time of healthy exposure cannot be recommended in this text, as the ozone layer varies in thickness throughout the world causing a wide variation in the ultraviolet ray Index from area to area. A local medical practitioner could give you advice on the maximum sun exposure times for your area.

Energy Outputs

As we take in measures of energy, we also expel or use various measures of energy in everything that we do in life. Our energy outputs are split into categories of physical and psychic energy outputs.

Psychic Energy

As the universe runs on various types of energy from the visible flame of a fire to the unseen flow of electrons, it only follows that we, as part of that universe, emit and use some of that unseen energy. Some of the psychic energy we generate is used in physical nerve impulses. Psychic energy is also used internally and expelled into our surroundings in the form of thinking and thought forms.

Physical Energy

We also expend physical energy in the basic form to keep our bodies operating, to have a heartbeat, to send nerve impulses through our body, to enjoy physical movement such as walking, running, etc. When our available energy is low, the physical output is the first to suffer in the form of feeling tired and lethargic. We require that our personal energy be at least of the level required to maintain our physical output to exist in this physical world.

All of the energy that we input into our body is processed and stored. Some of that energy is used for our body's operation for survival and maintenance. Anything that we do above the body's operation is used for the things that we choose to use the available energy for.

Energy Management

Our bodies are remarkable creations. For existence, in this world, they can adapt in a quite versatile manner to survive.

Once our bodies have made changes to suit their surroundings, they will attempt to exist within the restrictions of that environment, until our body accepts the new state as normal existence. This is why personal energy management is so important to our healthy survival.

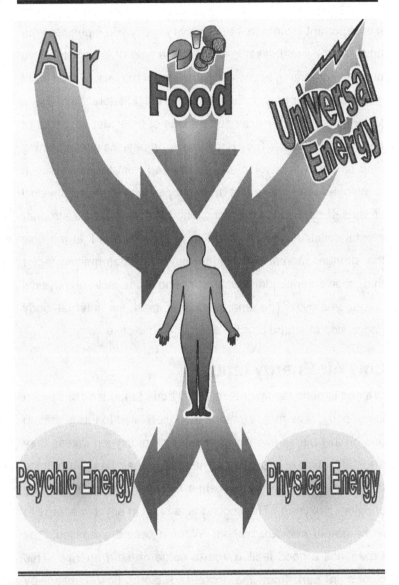

Figure 8.1 Energy Input Compared to Output

It is important to note that the type of energy you input into your body does not necessarily relate to the type of energy that you output. For example, you can supplement the lack of food input with psychic energy. East Indian Yogi Masters have been known to survive for extended periods of time with very little or no food and water. They can survive on physically maintaining their bodies with psychic energy inputted from the universe. It is also a well-known fact that people who survive physical ordeals of deprivation are ones who have displayed a stronger mental constitution. I would like to suggest that it is not only the stronger mental constitution that is the determining factor that supplements individuals suffering from lack of physical output energy. The energy comes from the internal body conversion of stored psychic energy to physical energy.

Low Air Energy Input

We can experience low mental acuity due to the lack of oxygen in our body. The most common thought related to this is that no one on this planet is afflicted with a lack of oxygen unless they are suffocating or drowning. The intake of air has two definite purposes. The first is to sustain life and purify the body by bringing in oxygen. The second is to bring in psychic energy to recharge our nervous system. When a person exercises, they experience a good feeling from a surge of extra energy. This comes in part from the increased blood flow caused by exercise. But the real cause of the euphoria is the increased breathing, where the body takes in oxygen at an increased pace. The extra air input increases blood purification. Also, the interaction with the electrons in the increased air volume intake within our lungs builds up the psychic energy level within the body. This is why athletes become addicted to exercise. A lot of the same benefits experienced by exercising can be achieved by using a discipline of deep breathing. One of the basic training disciplines of the Eastern mystics is called the science of breath. In this science, one learns how to breathe deeply and reap the benefits of enhanced health through increased blood oxygenation and additional psychic energy input. The way that you use the air about you is important in the quality of life. If you are low in psychic energy, exercise or do some deep breathing to re-energize yourself.

Low Psychic Energy Input

It also has been observed that some individuals with outstanding healing energy output have not balanced their psychic energy Input. While compensating for this energy imbalance with additional food energy Input, their bodies have converted a portion of the food input into psychic energy output. Unfortunately, a common by-product of this type of energy conversion is that the energy not expelled as psychic energy is stored in the form of physical body fat.

How many office workers who also suffer from the same lack of mental *(psychic)* energy supplement this shortage by boosting their overall energy input in the form of food that is high in caffeine and sugar so they can do their job. These office workers also will have the by-product of having the unused inputted physical energy in the form of food converted to body fat. Thus, we experience the mass overweight of people in the information era of our generation. One of the ways to gain a better psychic energy Input from the food input can be done by eating foods with a higher psychic energy value, such as raw vegetables and fruits. This will help to minimize the fat impact due to excessive eating. A better way to supplement your psychic energy input is with deep breathing or exercise.

Energy input versus energy output is one of the most important items that we need to learn to manage if we are going to be successful in having a healthy, successful lifestyle. It is important to manage your energy input of air, food, and psychic energies as compared to your outputs in the form of physical and psychic energies. If your current life conditions require the massive output of mental *(psychic)* energies, then I would suggest increasing your input of psychic energy in the form of meditation and deep breathing exercises. By doing this you will actively balance your input energy requirement as compared to the output energy being expelled. In the next chapter, we will explore techniques that can be used to build up our psychic energy Input. The danger of not increasing our psychic energy input when we sense our body is lacking psychic energy is that our body will gain the needed psychic energy any way it can. If your body is not trained to absorb psychic energy from the universe, it will attempt to rebalance energy content to gain that missing energy the only way it knows how, by eating! As everything contains electrons and has a certain amount of energy, universal psychic energy can be derived from the consumption of food. However, food contains chemical values in the form of calories, which also, if not expelled, will be stored in your body for future use in the form of fat. If this is the only way that you gather the psychic energy you need, you would have to counteract the eating with a vigorous exercise program to expel the extra physical energy that is being inputted in the form of food. I highly recommend that if you require extra psychic energy you learn and practice the techniques in the next chapter.

Low Food Energy Input

As well as physical problems, we can experience poor thought processes and low psychic output from the lack of food. That is why irritability and diets appear to go hand in hand. Before we talk of dieting, let us look at how our body operates with respect to food. Is your food input higher than your physical energy output? Food eaten is designed to give nutrients to the body. The quality of the food will result in the physical condition of your body. If you take in more food than you need, then your body will store the extra calories in the form of fat. If you eat less than your body requires, then you will suffer from the lack of nutrients required to live a healthy lifestyle. The volume of food required is one important factor to a healthy existence, but the other component is the quality of food consumed. In the computer industry, the term 'garbage in - garbage out' has been developed, which means that if bad information is entered into the computer, then the computer will give out bad information. Also, the computer files will get jammed up with bad information that can corrupt the computer memory and crash the entire computer system. The same concept can apply to our physical bodies. If we input low nutritional quality food into our body, some of that food will pass through our digestive system without adding any nutrients or energy to the body. But, as the computer can collect erroneous data, your body will pick up unhealthy food components and store them in the form of toxic fats. So it is just as important to measure the quality of the foods you eat as the quantity of your foods. I would like to suggest that a well-balanced diet be taken on which consists of a high portion of raw fruits, grains, and vegetables. It is important that you eat raw fruit and vegetables are low in fats and have the benefit of containing live energy since you are eating living matter. Grains contain nutrients and fibre that are used to clean our digestive system. The living energy of raw fruits and vegetables are also a source of psychic energy. When you cook fruits and vegetables, they lose the live energy and the inherent nutrients. As vegetables are processed for the supermarket, they also lose life energy and nutrients. A rule of thumb is, the more processing food has, the less nutritional value it has. In processed food, you can see labels that say Vitamin C enriched. This is done to replace nutrient value synthetically that was lost in the processing of that food. These are simple rules, but if you wish to gain more information about eating nutritiously, visit your local health food store.

The Energy Balancing Act

No matter how you do the math, the energy inputted into your body must equal your body's energy output. Since your body works on both physical and psychic energy, it is important to balance the input of food with the output of physical energy. It is also important to balance the input of and output of psychic energy. Only by managing and balancing these energies can you have a healthy lifestyle.

Energy Balancing Technique

Sit quietly in a chair with your eyes closed and visualize in your mind's eye, that you are in a shower of white light coming down from the sky above you, that is filling your body with energy. As the white light showers you, notice how the dull, tired feeling seems to disappear. Feel your body getting healthier. Let the energy shower flow relaxed energy into your physical body and relax. Do this until you relax and feel yourself breathing with little effort. Then slowly wake yourself with three deep breaths and then move as you feel comfortable to do.

Harnessing Psychic Energy

Energy Basics

We can do things that require more than our normal amount of universal psychic energy. Psychic healing, energizing a thought, building up our mental or physical constitution are some of the mental activities that use energy beyond our regular body needs. When we do these activities, we require getting the extra energy from somewhere. In some cases, psychic healers choose to share their personal energy with a sick or afflicted person and let their personal energy restore itself over a rest period. I do not recommend this, as a person giving out their energy depletes their personal psychic energy-level and, without a restoring technique, can experience feeling run down for an extended period of time after the energy sharing session. During this period of time, the reduced energy level will lower personal resistance to illness, resulting in a greater risk of becoming sick.

In this section, we will discuss a number of techniques that can be used based on various physical electrical models along with the benefits or restrictions of each method. We use electrical models as examples because electrical energy operates in a very similar manner to the Earth's energy field that we live in. The models drawn in the figures in this chapter can be used as visual focus points to aid in the use of psychic energy.

The Human Battery

In the electron theory, electrical energy can be induced through a chemical reaction in a battery. Electrons can flow through a wire, energizing a light when the switch is turned to the on position. One of the energy theories is that our body is made of chemicals and minerals. Thoughts and feelings are electrical impulses that our minds generate though internal chemical reactions within our bodies. If we can, through thought, influence the chemical makeup of our bodies to act as a psychic energy battery, we can then set up a potential charge in our bodies to create a psychic energy flow that can be used for healing ourselves and others. This energy can be used to energize ideas of what we want to happen in the future. This model of psychic energy control does work, and many people use it.

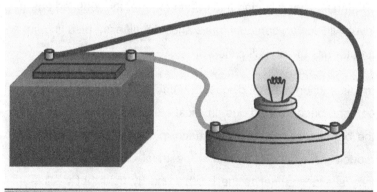

Figure 9.1 The Battery Technique

The one shortcoming of using the battery technique to move psychic energy by an internal chemical effect is that there is a limit to the amount of energy that you can handle at one time. An electrical battery is charged until the energy within it is used up. Then the battery needs recharging. A person who uses their internal energy supply in this way for psychic purposes will be like the battery that will be regularly depleted and continually require recharging. Recharging can be through sleeping, meditation, or eating. If not kept in check, this method of psychic energy transference can result in a cycle of overeating to achieve the extra chemical reaction to create psychic energy. The by-product can be extra calories and putting on extra weight.

The Psychic Generator

One of the more productive methods of producing electrical energy is by the use of a mechanical generator. Humankind uses mechanical generators powered by water, atomic energy, and wind. The generator principle is that the mechanical device converts physical energy by rotating the generator into movement of electrons through a wire. This is done through the use of electronic coils and magnetism.

Our bodies can generate psychic energy the same way a generator can produce electricity. This method of storing and using energy is based on the science of breath that is employed by Eastern society. The Eastern belief is based on the premise that the air is full of mystical energy, called prana. Since we breathe air into our lungs, it stands to reason that our lungs that extract oxygen can also extract the life force called prana out of that same breath of air. The electron theory supports this idea, as air that flows through the mouth, then the windpipe, and finally into our lungs creates friction. Where there is friction, there is a static electricity discharge. This discharge could be the natural electrical transference of electricity from the air around us to our bodies. Through the act of deep breathing, we can cleanse our bodies and energize them with this pranic energy. I would like to suggest that this pranic energy is universal psychic energy.

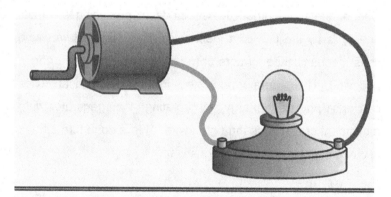

Figure 9.2 The Psychic Generator

The Western world, for the most part, tends not to believe in the use of pranic energy. The North American alternativo ic to exercise as a way of better well-being. The correlation between exercise and pranic energy has not been linked by many people in the exercise field. When we exercise, there are two basic things that we do. We increase our heart rate and our breathing rate. The Western world is more of a physical realm than a spiritual realm, so the belief is that increased heart rate is the reason people gain health benefits from the act of exercising. There are many accounts of exercising creating a state of well-being, a clearer mind, and a lower stress level. Exercising has been a real boon to better health in the world, but there are basic shortfalls to exercising. When a person exercises to raise their energy level, they can have the result of physically wearing out their body before its time and leaving themselves without possible means to renew their personal energy. As people age, they are less able to exercise, so they need to find an alternative means of generating psychic energy.

To address this situation, use exercise to keep your body in good physical condition and use deep breathing exercises to balance and refresh your psychic energy. Many stress therapists teach basic deep breathing techniques to patients suffering from stress. The technique is simply to, when under stress, take a deep breath to relax. By doing this, we are actually replenishing and balancing our personal psychic energy. When you feel out of balance or mentally stressed, take a moment to take about four deep breaths while standing or sitting as relaxed as you can be. It takes only a few seconds to do some deep breathing and release some of the tension in your body. This will build up your personal psychic energy when you are low. There are no side effects as in the previous techniques.

With practice of this technique, you can build up the duration time of the segments from three seconds to five seconds and the number of repetitions from three to five.

Breathing Exercise

Sit or stand quietly with your eyes closed. Take a deep breath. Inhale for 3 seconds. Hold the air in your lungs for 3 seconds. Exhale for 3 seconds. Pause for 3 seconds, then inhale for 3 seconds. Repeat this cycle 3 times.

Wind in Your Sail Technique

One of the most innovative mechanical devices that humankind has developed through the ages is the sailing ship. For centuries humankind has harnessed the wind and sailed the many seas and oceans of our physical world. If we look at the principle of harnessing and using the wind, we can apply the same principle to using psychic energy.

A sailing ship uses sails to capture the wind. Due to the size of a ship's sails, the amount of wind required to move the ship is very little. There is very little effort required to operate the sails and the rudder of the ship to capture and use the wind's energy. Collecting energy by sails does not create energy, but converts energy into motion. There is no fuel required to propel a sailing ship, making it a very energy-efficient tool for our use in the physical world.

As a ship's sails harness wind energy, we can harness psychic energy to achieve what we want to achieve in life. Psychic energy as electron energy happens to be around us all of the time. Just by the nature of the movement of the universe, universal psychic energy can naturally flow. All we have to do is direct the universal psychic energy flow for whatever we wish to use it for. This is the method that I prefer to handle universal psychic energy because, like using a sail and rudder of a sailing ship, we can direct the universal psychic energy without depleting our personal psychic energy resources as in the previous methods described.

By using the 'Wind Energy Technique', you can re-energize your mental and psychic energy quickly and easily without any side effects as in some of the previous exercises.

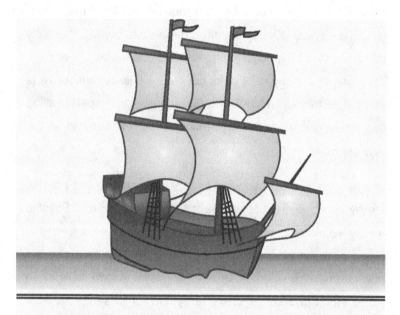

Figure 9.3 Wind in Your Sails Technique

Wind Energy Technique

Sit or stand quietly with your eyes closed. Take a deep breath. Relax, imagine that you are sitting in a lawn chair on a seashore and you can feel a soothing, warm breeze coming from behind you. This breeze is full of energy flowing from behind and slightly above your head, over you body to the ground. As you feel this breeze of energy flow, notice how you become more relaxed and energized. Relax and enjoy the energy breeze until you feel better. As you feel the breeze, you remember that, as a ship's sails collect wind as energy, you can use your body to collect energy. When you are ready, slowly wake yourself and enjoy the benefits of the energy shower.

Using Psychic Energy

Energy Use is Just a State of Mind

It is interesting to note that many of the religions of the world attribute the use of a god or universal energy source as a requirement for being able to have the ability to heal people and change outcomes of events. Prayer and meditation are used throughout the world in attempts to change unwanted results to desired outcomes. I would like to suggest that if prayer and meditation are used throughout the world, then there is a common link or factor that gives everyone their desired results. I would like to suggest that there is a common link that is more basic and simple than people realise.

The answer may lie in humankind's latent ability to actually mentally move electrons which are minutely present in everything that is physical. This idea may be closer to the truth than we think. When a person heals another, the patient feels a transfer of a non-measurable energy. This energy has been related to the rising of the Kundilini, the force, prana, ectoplasm, the god energy, universal energy, psychic energy, and life force, to name just a few. The list goes on and on, but there appears to be one thing in common, and that is, that there is recognition of an energy presence by many people. Some of us can command the use of that energy.

The effects of energy transference are present in many religions. The use of energy is also shrouded in ritual and mysticism. I find it interesting that many religious sects believe that they are the only ones that have the God-given right to use the universal energy that is all around us.

The use of universal psychic energy is just the way the physical universe operates. Healing and seeing the future in prophetic vision are more a religion than drug therapy, massage, herbal treatment, acupuncture, theoretical science, surgery, or any other form of healing or future speculation.

Everything that we do depends on the use of universal psychic energy. Anything that humanity has brought into existence has been a result of a thought that has been transferred into the physical world. We believe that physical action makes everything that we have come into existence. I would like to suggest that there is more to our existence than just doing things. There is a major distinction between animals and humans. That distinction is that we can imagine things, then use the thought energy to bring these items into existence. At this point, I am not discussing materializing items out of thin air, but transferring thoughts into physical matter to bring things into existence for our use. When Michelangelo carved the statue of David, he was asked 'how he could create such a magnificent sculpture?' His answer was 'David was always in the piece of stone, I just removed the parts that were not David'. This is a crude but accurate description how Humankind brings things into our 'Physical Realm' from the elusive World of thoughts and ideas.

When Michelangelo dreamed up the idea to make a statue of David, in his mind he could see David in every detail and believed that the image of David could be transferred from his thoughts to stone. Michelangelo's next task was to find the stone where the statue of David resided. Once the stone was found, all that remained was to chip away the parts of the stone that were not David. The process that Michelangelo used could be considered a crude method of materialization as it involved much personal physical effort.

This simple process is all it took. The process is simple but not easy. When I say simple, I mean anyone can do this. When I say not easy, I mean that it takes a great amount of mental energy and some physical energy to make the transition work.

Group Materialization

The industrialist, Andrew Carnegie used an interesting energy technique called the Master Mind Principle. This technique worked as a result of having a group of people sit together on a regular basis with the task of working toward a specific goal. By regular group sessions, the subconscious minds of the individuals would automatically link together causing a group intelligence to be formed, called the Master Mind. The Master Mind then became the driving force that would cause the goals of the group to move from the non-tangible idea realm into the physical realm that we live in. The use of the Master Mind Principle made Andrew Carnegie one of the richest men of his time. The people that worked in Carnegie's Master Mind Group also benefited from the Master Mind principle, as they also did quite well financially.

The Master Mind Principle is just one of the many variations of the use of the sea of universal energy' pool that we live in. The significant point of this concept is that it works without ritual or religious overtones. The process actually directs universal energy to create the setting needed to cause an event to occur. The very same principle is used in various religious groups' healing ceremonies. Churches employ this technique in group prayer, where a number of people congregate to focus prayer for the healing of one individual. Through group prayer to their Divinity, a positive result is achieved. To be effective, prayer groups usually work with everyone at the same location at the time of prayer. This keeps everyone in tune with or of like mind of what they are praying for.

There is also another twist to this system of creating Master Mind results, which is when prayer groups decide in advance to pray for a specific item at a specific time. No matter where the individuals are at the specified time, they stop and pray. The results are the same. The Master Mind effect takes over, and positive results are achieved. All the same principles used in prayer groups are but a variation of the ones used in the Master Mind Groups.

I would like to suggest that both religious and non-religious groups are using the same basic energy transfer techniques to achieve a desired result. Both employ very different methods, one ritualistic and one non-ritualistic, with both getting observable results. This would suggest that the factor that causes the results is not a specific religion but the use of universal energy. I do believe that the principle holds true for the way the Universe that we live in operates, but I also believe that belief in a supreme being can significantly enhance the results. Personal beliefs and religious beliefs are not the topic of this book. I would suggest that the reader use these natural laws as they see fit and fit these ideas into their personal beliefs. Remember, the use of universal energy is the same as using electricity. There are no religious conflicts with electricity, so there should be no conflicts with using universal energy. At this point, I will leave the religious aspects of using universal energy to the reader's belief system, as this book is not addressing theological issues.

The operation of the Master Mind system does have serious repercussions for us in society as a result of our culture. We have all seen religious shows on television where the speaker asks all the viewers to pray about one item for a good purpose. Through the linking of global telecommunications, people throughout the world can link together at one time in a powerful use of the Master Mind technique. People throughout the world can now energize one idea to make a positive change in the world for humankind. This use of global technology is a double-edged sword. There can be good achieved, or through the absent-minded use of the same medium there can be great energy amassed to destructive events. When a large viewing audience is watching a violent television program, the group intelligence unknowingly creates a version of the Master Mind to achieve the goals of the television program. With the current level of violence on television, this should be of great concern to all of us.

The group intelligence technique does work in bringing things from the idea realm to the physical realm that we live in. The technique still requires physical action to make the transfer complete. Materialization at this level sets the stage for events to happen for the manifestation of events or physical items from the idea realm to the physical realm. To make the actual transition complete, someone is required to take physical action that starts the chain of events to bring a change or a physical item into existence. If there is one place we fall short of manifesting what we want, it is the lack of physical action to start the chain of events in the physical realm. This is where many of us fall short of actually achieving the goals that we set out to achieve in our lives.

When I talk to people or groups that prayed or energized an event to happen and did not get results, it reminds me of the story of the man who drowned in the flood. The story goes as follows.

There once was a flood where a man climbed to the roof of his house to escape the water. The water was all about him, and there was no way to escape as the waters rose. He was a religious man, so he prayed to God for deliverance from the waters that day and waited for a miracle to happen. As he waited, two boys came by in a canoe and offered to take him to shore. He turned down their offer and said that his God would deliver him from the flood. The waters rose. A man came in a motorboat and offered to save the man on the roof, but the reply was the same. He turned down the offer and said that his God would deliver him from the flood. The waters rose. Soon the water was almost to the tip of the roof and a helicopter came and offered to save the man from certain doom. The man's faith did not waver; his reply was the same. He turned down the offer and said that his God would deliver him from the flood. The waters rose and the man eventually was swept away and drowned. Upon drowning, he found himself at the Gates of Heaven. Upon the man's arrival at Heaven's Gate, Saint Peter said," What are you doing here? It was not your time to die!" The man replied, "I don't know. I prayed for deliverance and God did not save me." Saint Peter said, "That is really strange. I sent a canoe, a motor-boat, and a helicopter to save you. Did they not arrive in time?"

This little story does signify how we can actually set up the universal psychic energy to bring an event to pass and not recognize the result when we are face to face with it. If we do not recognise the transfer point from the idea realm to the physical realm and take action, the result we desire will not occur. In the case of the story, the man prayed and believed that his prayer would be answered, but he did not take the simple action of accepting a ride. But for the lack of recognition that his prayer was answered and the fact that all he had to do was to accept the ride from the boat, canoe or the helicopter, he would have survived the flood. The same holds true in our lives. All we have to do is to take that small physical action to bring something into existence in the physical realm". Many times all it takes is a small physical act to unleash the universal psychic energy' into the world for the purpose it is gathered for.

That story is much like how many people envision their prayers, meditations, and dreams being answered. To bring things out of the idea realm to the physical realm it takes some physical effort to complete the cycle. In the story, the man prayed, his prayers were answered, but he did not recognize that he had to take the small physical step to bring his prayer into reality! How many things do we pray for or energize for but pass up the opportunity when everything we need for success is within our grasp?

The Power to Heal

Healing and Religion

I do support that faith in a supreme being will bring miraculous healing results. If you have faith in a particular religious icon, by all means use that faith as it works for you. But I also believe that the same results are possible through the use of techniques unique to the laws of physics and the transfer of energy. Healing is possible without complicated religious ceremonies.

All true healing results from an application of perfectly natural laws, and the power employed is as natural as electricity. I would like to suggest that the previously discussed universal psychic energy is the tool that we use for healing. In many of the world's religions, there are healing practitioners that heal people using similar energy techniques. No matter what technique or religion is used, successful healing results are achieved all over the planet. The ability to heal is not only residing in the human brain but is distributed through every cell in your body. Each and every cell in your body contains some mind energy that links it with every other cell in your body as part of your mind. Whether these cells are of bone, blood, or tissue, they are connected with universal psychic energy and are subject to thoughts that suggest a level of health. These cells can respond and make that level of health a reality.

Healing Methods

There are many methods of healing that are used throughout the world. All of the methods work because of the use of the energy field that we live in. The energy field supplies the material needed for healing, and the healing method used is the practitioner's chosen tool used to heal the patient. All healing methods work in a slightly different manner, but all methods take the energy about us and redistribute it into the person being healed. The component that makes people healing people possible is the directing of the universal psychic energy around us with our personal energy. This component is the common link to make all of the following techniques possible.

Laying on of Hands

Laying on of hands is a popular method of Christian healing. The technique works because the people in the room are sharing thoughts of healing. The thoughts allow a practitioner or a number of participants to touch the patient, causing the transfer of universal psychic energy from them to the patient. Once it is received, the patient's body then uses the energy to enhance its natural healing ability.

Prayer Circles

Prayer circles are effective because a group of people congregate in one location and share one specific thought, that is, the healing of a specific patient. The shared thought directs the universal psychic energy to the patient's body, enhancing that person's natural healing ability.

Pranic Healing

Pranic healing is where the concentrating of the universal psychic energy around us to an affected part of a body results in healing to occur. This method directs universal psychic energy, with or without physical contact, to the person being healed. Prana is recognized by Eastern philosophy as the inherent energy that surrounds us that can be directed. Pranic healing is very similar to the Western method of laying on of hands, which is documented in the Bible. Some Christian sects continue to practice laying on of hands as a method of healing.

Mental Healing

Mental Healing is where the practitioner sends mental thoughts to the sick person's mind until it responds to the thought. The response to the new thought pattern allows the afflicted person's mind to create the actual healing. This method appears to be similar to methods that employ a prayer to aid a patient in their healing. In Eastern philosophy, the practitioner goes into meditation and envisions the person to be healed being healed. By doing this in a meditative state, the universal psychic energy that surrounds us is mentally directed to the person to be healed. A Western technique that is used is absent prayer, where a prayer group will pray for a sick person who may be in a hospital. The group prayer directs energy to the sick person, who can use the energy for personal healing.

Spiritual Healing

Spiritual Healing is where a person on a higher spiritual level transfers a thought to a less evolved being, who is healed due to the enlightenment of a new concept. This is probably the way Jesus accomplished his many miracles of healing.

Other methods of instantaneous spiritual healing occur when a person becomes enlightened to a spiritual truth. That allows that person to instantly drop the belief that caused a physical illness. This works because any spiritual growth brings us closer to God and frees us from some of the shackles and limitations of the physical realm we live in.

Transference Healing

A powerful and interesting method of healing is through the method of thought transference. This technique differs from the other methods of healing in that it is the only method where transference of universal psychic energy is not the only element of the cure. In this method, the practitioner projects to the patient the thought of how a healthy body is to be. The patient's body then receives the thought and uses it as a map to adjust and heal itself. This method works in the same way that psychologists heal mentally ill patients. Just as planting thought seeds of how to have a better life can change a person's outlook and ability to cope in life, planting the same seeds into a person's subconscious mind will allow them to heal themselves just as easily.

This type of mental connection is apparent in the healing performed almost effortlessly by the East Indian gurus. With no apparent ritual, a guru can make an instantaneous healing occur. For them it is easy, because their years of training allow them to very quickly drop into their subconscious minds. From the subconscious mind, the guru commands a portion of universal energy to move from one place to another. Along with the energy, the guru places a vision of pure health into the patient's subconscious mind. The implanted energy in the patient's body for healing is then productively used by the patient's subconscious mind for healing. The subconscious mind's analytical nature will instantly use the energy as directed and make the healing occur. The patient's body will respond by accepting the healing directions and hence become healed of any infirmity.

The pure health vision, once implanted in the patient's subconscious mind and accepted, then acts as a part of our internal universal map for using the universal psychic energy field about us for an effective healing and to maintain a good level of health in the future.

Amulet Healing

Amulet healing is a system of powerful cure and protection for the believers of amulet power. Amulet power is based on two things: personal belief in the power of a symbol and the group belief throughout the world of the symbol's power. If you believe that an amulet will bring you personal luck, the amulet acts as a focus point for your belief. Others that believe that the particular amulet sign has power also share this thought. Belief is a thought energy that can direct the universal psychic energy around us to create the circumstances to bring a thought into the physical realm. An amulet's power come from the number of people alive who believe in what the Amulet can do. The belief in the symbol links the believers in a single energy chain, which gives the symbol on the Amulet the power to heal. The greater the group of believers, the stronger the Amulet. This is why Amulets that are not popular appear to have little or no power as compared to the popular symbols.

Colour Therapy

Colour therapy is a very straightforward method of healing. Each colour reflects a hue of light. What we actually see is the part of the light spectrum that the colour does not absorb. The reflection is light energy of a specific frequency. We are actually bathing in the colour that we see. Along with that colour flows some universal psychic energy that is modified by the frequency of the light. Colour therapy is a slow process that works. We choose colours for our surroundings based on what feels comfortable. Imagine what would happen if we chose colours for our homes to enhance the way we wish to be. Use of colours to harness universal psychic energy is a subtle but powerful tool that anyone can use.

Healing with Stones

Healing with stones is a method of healing that is simple to use. Stones are minerals that are composed of chemicals much like our bodies. Contact with stones can cause a chemical exchange. Some of the vitamins we use are minerals. Alchemists of old would actually grind up minerals and have people swallow them for various cures. As most minerals can conduct or insulate from heat and electrical energy, it follows that they can also conduct or insulate universal psychic energy. Since all minerals contain different molecular structures, they will collect and transfer different frequencies of universal psychic energy. Crystal mineral structures such as quartz, amethyst, and citrine can amplify the subtle universal psychic energy in the surrounding area. Placement of crystals in the area of where you reside can enrich the energy atmosphere that you live in.

Aromatherapy

Aromatherapy is a healing method where one inhales aromas from herbal oils or burning herbs to enhance one's health. The aromas can carry the medicinal ingredients through the air. We then breathe the air, and the medicinal ingredients are quickly transferred into our body through the lungs. As the herbs are denser than the air, they have a higher ability than air to collect universal psychic energy. Besides gaining the healing properties from the medicinal ingredients, you also benefit from the additional universal psychic energy that you inhale. Some of the herbal aromas have greater ability than others to enhance the flow of universal psychic energy into our bodies.

God and Healing

In many of the healing disciplines, reliance on healing is given to God or a supreme being. It is interesting to note that faith in a higher being strengthens healing abilities and is usually associated with the healer's interest in spiritual growth. All energy transfer and healing methods will work on the basis of controlling energy transference, but it has been shown to be more effective when the healer has a strong personal spiritual belief that they live by. Belief in a higher source of intelligence and energy seems to link us not only to the energy of the Earth, but also to a source of spiritual knowledge that will change and influence our personal beliefs and abilities. It is no coincidence that people with high spiritual belief structures have naturally more healing abilities than those that have a low level of personal faith. Belief in God or a being in tune with the spiritual side of the universe also can have the benefit of a higher level of general health and stronger longevity factor in this physical life.

My recommendation to anyone who wishes to go into the healing field is to build a solid personal spiritual belief structure that is as strongly held as any factual thought that they possess. Only when you are secure in where you fit in the universe, both physically and spiritually, can you become mentally free to exercise control over the things that we cannot see or measure by conventional scientific methods.

Disassociation from God can result with various levels of illness. Being in tune with God does give the result of good health. The common link of many religions is that there is a supreme being that is the controlling force that everything that exists depends on. God has many names, from names of personage to that of the God Force. This leads us to the point where God and the subtle energy about us are linked in some way.

Faith and Healing

Faith to recognise the existence of universal psychic energy and that it works and achieves results is a challenge for many. Ancient humankind used universal psychic energy as needed for healing and energizing things that they could not explain or control by conventional means. As universal psychic energy could not be scientifically proven, the scientific community rejected it. This did not deter the religious community of the world; universal psychic energy was embraced and successfully used by many religions. The use of universal energy in religious practice complemented the idea that faith will give future results. Faith does not require scientific proof for the observed results achieved by the use of universal psychic energy, so the only reasonable explanation for the effect of healing was that healing was a result of faith. Scientists are still very reluctant to attempt to dispute faith, as it is another scientifically unproven commodity. This fit into the natural progression of faith in God or a supreme being, the premise being: **'IF WE CANNOT PROVE GOD'S EXISTENCE, BUT WE BELIEVE HE EXISTS, THEN WE CAN BE HEALED BY FAITH.'** By putting these two premises together, many religions built the fact that healing is due to the belief in God. So if we believe and meditate on the Lord, we can be healed. The system works with good results.

The Law of Attraction

Basically, the law of attraction is explained as, what you concentrate on the most is what the mental forces around you will bring into your physical reality. So, if you concentrate on illness, you will be sick as a result. If you concentrate on excellent health as a result of your thoughts, you will attain excellent health. If you concentrate on being poor, you will attain that result. If you put your mental energies to achieving one goal at a time, your thoughts will permeate the energy field that you live in, and that energy will act the same way as a transmitter does to a homing beacon. What you put into the energy field around you will attract to you the circumstances to make the opportunities, to herald events into your life that make the thoughts a reality.

Repetitive Healing Syndrome

You may then ask what causes the repetitive healing syndrome, where a patient gets healed, observable changes are seen, but the effect soon wears off and the patient again regains his or her illness. Did the healing really occur, or was the person duped? In the case of real metaphysical healing, this can be easily explained as follows: The patient maintains a low energy level based on his or her beliefs and suffers from the lack of active use of their subconscious mind. That person then does not have the ability to draw from the universal energy field to attain excellent health. When a healing occurs, the patient is infused with energy that will maintain a good state of health until the energy is depleted. As the infused universal psychic energy is used up, the patient's illness returns. The patient then returns for another healing. What the patient is actually doing is returning for another boost of universal psychic energy, the same as recharging a battery that has run down.

During, a healing the patient is charged with universal psychic energy. The effectiveness of the healing is dependent on the practitioner's command of the universal energy field. The greater the command, the greater the results. The second component of the healing is the subconscious mind transference of the healthy state of being and the thought pattern to maintain a healthy energy flow. For some people, the thought transference can happen on the first healing, while for others, two or three healing sessions may be required, and yet for others, the thought transference never happens. These are the people that spend their lives running from healer to healer looking for another energy fix.

But those that accept the healing energy, along with the subconscious thought pattern of good health, comes the enjoyment of a new lifestyle of health. They may experience the cure of something as small as an allergy to something as miraculous as the disappearance of a cancerous growth forever.

Common Link in all Methods of Healing

There is a common link among the spiritual healers, the gurus of India, the Shaolin of Asia, the psychic healers of the world, and the Christian healers of North America. The link is that they all use their subconscious minds to attain results.

Although the above thoughts lead many religions to believe that they have the sole magic healing package, I believe that in using the techniques in this text you will get results no matter what your particular religious faith is. This healing training can be done without the overtures of any specific religion or faith rituals.

All non-medical healers do some things that are in common, which gives the similar results as shown in the following table.

Conditions for Healing Results

There are many factors that cause healing to work or not to work. Healing results depend on the following:

- *The patient's belief structure. If a patient believes that he/she will receive a healing, that person will receive their healing. A person with a high belief coupled with a highly skilled practitioner can experience miraculous results. A person with a low level of belief will get poor or no healing results. Even if the practitioner has the ability to move mountains, he/she cannot heal a person who rejects the healing, and very little or nothing will happen.*

- *The practitioner's command of the universal energy field. The greater the practitioner's command of universal psychic energy, the greater are the achievable results in healing.*

Conditions for Healing Results (continued)

- *Subconscious thought transference must happen for the healing to become permanent. A dramatic healing happens as a result of the inflicted person's mind responding to and taking on the practitioner's thought patterns of good health along with the universal psychic energy transfer. The inflicted person then has his/her map of the universe modified so that their subconscious mind has an internal reference of excellent health to control the physical and mental being in that person's life. Subconsciously, the individual is healed; then the outward physical manifestations of health take place.*

Physical Methodology for Healing

We as physical beings are conduits for the flow of universal psychic energy in the same way a wire transfers electrical energy. Different types of electrical wires conduct electrical energy with different levels of efficiency. All living things also conduct universal psychic energy at different levels of efficiency. The difference between humans and electrical wire is that in energy conduction a wire will never change its efficiency level for handling electricity, but through training humans can improve their efficiency level for conducting universal psychic energy.

A wire is physically connected to an electrical source to enable it to conduct electricity. As conductors of universal psychic energy, we are connected to our source of energy, which is the Earth's energy field. Universal psychic energy is all about us, the same way that fish in a pond are surrounded by and in contact with water. We live in and are in contact with the universal psychic energy field at all times, making it readily available for instant use. Awareness of this constant contact with universal psychic energy is not apparent to most people, as we are constantly in contact with this energy.

If there is a lack of universal psychic energy around you, you are immediately aware of it. An example of an area where you will experience a lack of universal psychic energy is in a hospital's cancer ward. The moment you enter this area, you can feel a distinct lack of energy or the feeling of life about you. The people in this place have lost their ability to draw universal energy for physical survival. You also may experience a draining feeling just by being there.

If you then enter a psychiatric ward of the same hospital, you will have an uneasy feeling. This is brought about by the way the people in that ward scramble the universal energy around them.

Some people that visit psychiatric wards actually have their personal energy field scrambled so badly that they may behave as an escaped patient for a few days until the effect wears off.

When you go into a wooded area or a garden, you can feel very relaxed and at peace from the high level of the universal energy flowing through the living plants about you. Plants are known to be abundant with an unknown energy. This energy can be photographed using Kirlian photography. Even if a part of a plant is removed, the energy imprint of the removed part can still be seen in a Kirlian photograph taken after the part is removed. An area full of plants is an excellent place to recharge your personal energy within your body when you feel energy depleted. That is why forest resorts and cabins are relaxing to be in.

As illustrated in the above examples you can see or feel the inconsistencies in the universal energy field. In a place where people are dying there is a definite lack of universal energy as compared to a forest that is fully abundant with universal energy. Focus on being aware of these differences and you will have taken the first step to mastering the use of the universal energy field in healing.

Common Link in All Methods of Healing

- *Both healer and patient believe that healing can occur.*

- *All healers strive for spiritual enlightenment.*

- *Healers operate their healing out of the unseen realm of faith, faith that if they follow a certain ritual or use a certain technique, they will attain a healing result.*

- *Healers experience the feeling of the flow of the universal energy, either around them or through them. Some of the names attached to this have been the power of God, the power of the spirit, prana, psychic power, psychic energy, and my favourite, universal psychic energy, just to name a few.*

Common Link in All Methods of Healing (continued)

- *All healers delve deeply into some form of spiritual thought. These thoughts spur the imagination, which is the tool that operates the subconscious mind. By exercising this tool, thought patterns are established that give the healers a more direct access to the subconscious mind.*

- *Healers gain access to the universal energy field without knowing the science of how or why they have gained this access. This is why various religions put a sole claim on healing.*

- *Each religion that uses healing as a part of their doctrine believes that their regimen of faith has caused the healing to occur.*

- *Patients believe they feel some immediate change during the healing ceremony.*

The Healing Technique

Natural Energy Flow

There is a natural energy flow from the atmosphere around you through your body to the ground below you. This flow happens due to the electron field that we live in as discussed in earlier chapters. The natural energy flow is shown in Figure 12.1.

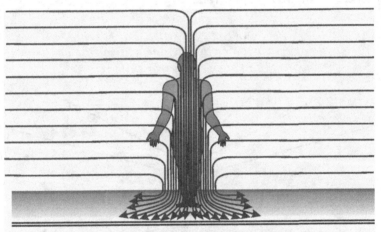

Figure 12.1 The Natural Energy Flow

Contact with another person causes a mix of energy between the two people. The natural energy flows through both of the people to the Earth below. If there is an absence of conscious energy control, a natural mixing of personal energy happens between both individuals. This natural energy makes it easy to pick up an energy pattern from another person you are in

145

physical contact with. This natural mix can also allow you to be able to transfer an energy pattern to another individual either subconsciously or consciously. Healing can be done by either physically contacting or not contacting a person to transfer energy. Since we are conductors of energy, we can direct this natural flow of energy through our body from the air around us and direct that energy through our body and finally out of our hands, as shown in Figure 12.2.

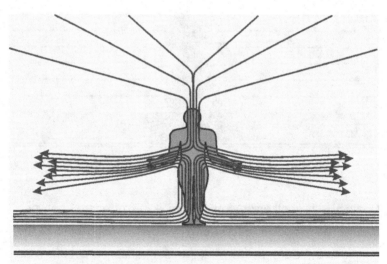

Figure 12.2 Directing Universal Psychic Energy

Personal Healing for Good Health

- *Find a quiet, comfortable place where you will not be disturbed.*

- *Sit or lie down, whichever makes you feel more comfortable.*

- *Close your eyes and breathe deeply. With each breath, feel the tension in your body slowly flowing out through your toes and fingertips.*

- *Once relaxed, imagine a ball of white light above your head. Feel this white light shining on you, filling you with a feeling of comfortable warmth and well-being. As the white light flows in, you sense the old darker colored energy flowing out of your body into the earth below.*

- *Continue this process until your body is full of the energizing white light energy.*

- *Once your body is full of the white light energy, you can either have a restful sleep or waken feeling re-energized.*

Personal Pin Point Healing

- *Find a quiet, comfortable place where you will not be disturbed.*

- *Sit or lie down, whichever makes you feel more comfortable.*

- *Close your eyes and breathe deeply. While breathing deeply, imagine that all the tension in your body is slowly flowing out through your toes and fingertips.*

- *Once you are relaxed you will notice that above you is a ball of white light. Imagine that this white light is shining upon you like a narrow flashlight beam of warm, comfortable energy. As the white light flows in you sense that the old, darker colored energy in your body is flowing out toward the Earth, where it will be re-energized.*

- *Continue this process until the spot in your body that you wanted to energize is full of the energizing white light energy.*

- *Once done, you can either have a restful sleep or waken feeling re-energized.*

Energy Healing

To perform a healing is a matter of redirecting the universal psychic energy about you by the use of your imagination. All that you have to do is to close your eyes and imagine that you are surrounded by a mass of infinite energy of bright, vibrant colours. Due to the fact that you are using your subconscious mind and your imagination, you will imagine the energy and its flow in a different way than anyone else. This is fine. As you imagine the energies, see them slowly swirling above you and then coming down through you. As you raise your right arm, imagine the energy flowing down through your body and out of your arm. As you do this, feel the exhilaration of the energy flow and the warm feeling associated with being full of this energy, as a conduit transferring electricity. Once you have transferred energy through you, the next step is to imagine the flow to stop and once the flow is stopped make sure that you fill yourself with energy to maintain your personal well-being. Before attempting to heal another person, you must first be proficient in this energy transfer procedure.

Once you can use your imagination to start the energy flow and stop the energy flow, you are then ready to move on to the next step, a personal healing. This is done by simply making the energy transfer as in the last procedure, but instead of having the energy flow out of your right arm, you can put your right hand on an afflicted part of your body and transfer the energy there. While you are making the energy flow, imagine in your mind the vision of yourself being in perfect health. Do this energy transfer until the picture of perfect health in your mind feels real. At this point you can stop the energy flow and enjoy a better level of health. With practice, you can reach the level where you will be able to put yourself into a state of perfect health. An advanced variation of this technique is to simply transfer the universal psychic energy to an illness affected body part by imagining that the energy flow is absorbed from around you and goes into your body directly to that afflicted part. Once either variation of this technique is mastered, you are ready to move on to the next step, to facilitate the healing of another person.

Healing Others

To heal another person, the technique is basically the same as healing yourself. The difference is that instead of filling yourself with universal psychic energy, you fill the other person with the universal psychic energy. To do this, imagine the person in your mind and then, with them in your mind, create the energy flow. Imagine that person in perfect health and visualize him or her being filled with the universal psychic energy. When the vision appears of that person in perfect health full of universal psychic energy, the healing is complete. At this point stop the flow of energy and disconnect the image of the person from your mind. Make sure that you fill yourself with the universal psychic energy, and then you are finished the healing. A healing of this nature can be done by physically contacting the person to be healed. This type of healing also can be done without touching the person being healed. As a matter of fact, healing can be done through the universal energy field with no limitation of distance between the practitioner and the patient.

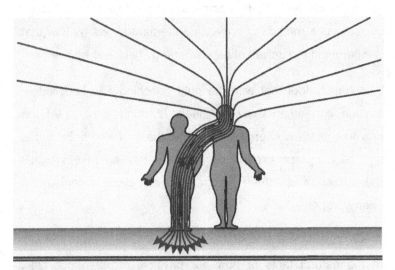

Figure 12.3 The Natural Universal Psychic Energy Flow

In a nutshell, the above is all that is necessary to heal yourself or another person. The system is simple. Note: I stated the system is simple, not easy. To master the technique does take some time. For some people, the learning period may be a few days, for others a few years. The variables in mastering the technique are the person's ability to visualize in his or her imagination the energy flow, the ability to feel the energy flow about them, and the ability to visualize an internal picture of good health.

Using this method of healing does not involve personal invasion of spirit. This method also involves no risk of personal injury to you or the person that the energy is directed to. This technique basically is a method of enhancing the natural energy flow that is inherent in the universal psychic energy field that we live in.

I personally feel that with the right coaching and knowledge, anyone can attain excellent health through the use of the universal psychic energy field around them. I also believe that anyone can also experience excellent healing results within themselves and others using this very basic technique of energy transfer.

Again, I would like to repeat that this energy transfer is just one of the natural facts of how our physical universe operates. Personal and religious beliefs can enhance the healing effects but are not necessary to have the effect occur. The more that you practice healing with this natural energy, the more proficient you will become at using the energy.

Directing Healing Energy to Another Person

- *Find a quiet, comfortable place where you will not be disturbed.*

- *Have the patient sit or lie down, whichever makes the patient feel more comfortable.*

- *Have the patient close their eyes and breathe deeply to relax. Guide the patient through one of the relaxation techniques from this book.*

- *Once the patient is relaxed, you can start the treatment.*

- *Close your eyes; visualize a ball of white light above you. Imagine that this white light is shining upon you and the patient like a spotlight.*

- *In your imagination, see the light flowing down upon you and the patient. Direct that light from above through the patient.*

Directing Healing Energy to Another Person *(continued)*

- *Once the white light washes any perceived dark blotches away from the patient's body, the treatment is complete.*

- *Tell the patient that 'where the white light touches you, it fills the point it is shining on with a comfortable, warm feeling. As the white light flows in, you sense that the old, darker colored energy in your body is flowing out toward the Earth, where it will be re-energized.'*

- *Once done, gently guide the patient in a gentle voice to wakefulness using suggestions to awaken and feel fully refreshed.*

- *Allow the patient a few minutes to regain full consciousness.*

One final thought on healing is that I recommend an ill person does not attempt to heal another. There are sound reasons for this. First of all, if you are ill, you are not balancing your internal energies in a normal manner. You may deplete your personal energy store and unbalance the other person's energy to also complicate their health situation. If you attempt to heal them, you may also unconsciously send them an imprint of your ill health to complicate their healing process, as they can take on the image of your illness with the energy received for the healing.

If you are ill, ask someone else to do the healing or pray for a healing for that sick person to remove the chance of transferring your illness.

Resistance to the Natural Laws

Limiting Thoughts

The statements in this book can have some very profound repercussions on the way that we view religions, cults, medicine, physics, and healing rituals. Many centuries of religious ritual and religious writings now can be evaluated with new eyes. Just think of how man's thoughts of the universe changed when Galileo, through the use of a telescope, mapped the universe and proved that the Earth rotated about the Sun. Just talking of these scientific discoveries labelled Galileo as being a heretic. Everyone in the Christian world at that time knew that the Sun rotated about the Earth. This theology was established on the premise that man was God's ultimate creation and, being so, man would be placed in the centre of the universe. Therefore, it was logical that man's home, the Earth, could be set only in the centre of the universe. Due to this summation of knowledge up to Galileo's discovery, the Earth must be at the centre of the universe and everything else in the universe must rotate about man's home, Earth. Any thinking otherwise was just plain religious heresy. Anyone who believed anything different was considered a heretic attacking the divine existence of an all-powerful God. For Galileo to have his contemporaries accept his research as scientific fact, Galileo was expected to prove that God did not exist. Through the years, we have come to accept Galileo's theories and emotionally accept the fact that our home, Earth, rotates around the Sun. The fact that the Earth rotates about the Sun has not lessened our value of God in man's personal religious value system.

I expect that a negative response to the information in this text can be expected from some religions and members of the scientific and medical communities. Various religious viewpoints on healing range from, any healing other than medical healing does not exist, to their specific religion's healing methods being, in the eyes of God, the only divine approved method of healing available.

Could you imagine presenting this paper to a religious group which believes that healing using universal psychic energy is just a form of trickery and the result of being in league with dark forces of a highly negative nature? How could you logically get these people to acknowledge these findings? How could you even present a case that would make them listen? Their fears are that if they were to listen to such heresy, they would surely lose their immortal souls. These people just would not listen.

On the other end of the religious scale are those religions that practice a ritualistic healing that does achieve results. If you were to try to sell these findings to them, they would acknowlodge that healing based on physical laws can occur, but they probably would not openly show any agreement, the reason being that, to accept that healing has no religious or mystical connections would invalidate one of their religion's basic cornerstones. If they lost the converts that joined the flock for religious healing, their religion would surely suffer. Because of this political fact these religions could not support healing with universal psychic energy, as it would undermine their very existence.

Those Who Heal

The picture of people being healed through a simple application of existing physical laws and a standard healing technique is not as bleak as it appears. Although there is much resistance from the religious communities, there are many people out there who could very easily use these healing techniques; many of them would be doing it out of basic need for better health. Eventually, people will learn how the natural physical laws of universal psychic energy work and put them into practice. As society gets more and more technically competent, people will question many of the cornerstones of belief currently held as indisputable ground. At this time, the distinction of universal psychic energy, God, and religion can be separated. People will come to realize that when Jesus walked the Earth, he demonstrated in a human form what humankind could do. Jesus did not regard the miracles as a religion. He just used the universal psychic energy to heal people he took pity upon. Jesus' real mission here was to teach us Christianity, but somehow humanity focused on the physical healing and lost the principle behind a lot of his religious teachings. Once this realization is made, man can move on and enjoy healing as a part of normal life activities without religious ritual. Humankind at that time will also have some of the mystical dogma removed from religion so that the true meaning of religion can be studied.

The Healing Revolution

The evolution to widespread use of universal psychic energy healing will eventually happen, if not as a result of this research, as a result of mental evolution. There is one other thing that will happen that will all of a sudden bring to the forefront the simplicity of healing with universal energy and make it a new medical technology. This will be when some scientist can perfect a device that will measure universal energy. Once mechanical means exist of proving universal psychic energy, it will take a very short period of time to measure the effect of psychic healing and to quantify the existence of universal psychic energy. Once a mechanical measuring device is created, healing with universal psychic energy will become an indisputable fact.

Once the universal psychic energy method of healing is quantified, standard healing techniques can be put into place.

Then whole medical and drug industries around the world will be greatly impacted. The need for drugs will diminish. The drug companies will have to change their markets to a preventative herbal industry. Practitioners, without the need for anaesthetics or post-operation drug therapy, will cure sickness. Hospitals will also drastically change. Many diseases that require a long stay in the hospital will then be treated as outpatient therapy, or the treatment may even be done by a family member at no medical charge. Hospitals would then greatly reduce in size, as the only real function that they would serve is to operate on people who have suffered a physical trauma and require immediate medical intervention. The intervention would be in the form of setting broken bones and sewing up lacerations from accidents.

When we can definitively measure and use universal psychic energy, it will change the total way the world society handles sickness and pain. Healing will be done without any side-effects. Total health will become a person's goal, as it will become so easy to achieve. The world economy will change as a result of the lower medical and drug administration needs. Truly the day will come when universal psychic energy healing will be a reality. The only question is when will the use of the universal energy become a viable scientific technology? When will this energy technology become available as alternative healing practice in the medical community?

Until then, such persons as you will be the pioneers in this new methodology in healing.

Future Challenges

Healing Today

Through the centuries, many religions have claimed healing as part of their religious theologies. In fact, many faiths claim that only their religion is the one and true source of divine healing. These religions usually accompany their healing method with a complicated ritual that has, through the years, become the standard for the followers to obey if they want to have divine intervention for an illness and the attainment of good health. If for some reason a healing does not occur, it is simply written off as not being in the will of God.

Although healing is incorporated in many religions, the process of healing is not dependent on religious rituals. Healing and the observable effects can be attributed to natural physical laws. Healing is dependent on the use of universal psychic energy. The director of this energy is the subconscious mind. The working of universal psychic energy is very similar to the working of electricity. Universal psychic energy and electricity are two unseen forces that deliver an effect. The only difference between universal psychic energy and electricity is that we can mechanically measure electricity. Although we do not understand how electricity really works, we accept it as factual because we can measure it. To date there is no real way to mechanically measure universal psychic energy. Without a definitive mechanical measurement of universal psychic energy, the scientific community will not accept its existence. However the problem that the scientific community has is that the results of universal psychic energy can be observed in healing and, although discounted, cannot be dismissed. The only exception is that universal energy can be used as a healing enhancement, not a replacement for your medical professional.

Healing Technology of Tomorrow

By accessing the subconscious mind, we can access the limitless field of universal psychic energy and heal others or ourselves by using simple techniques. No religious ceremonies with the proper training are required. Universal psychic energy can be used in healing as easily as turning on a light switch. Healing with universal psychic energy is simply the transfer of energy to an inflicted person along with the thought patterns of abundant health. Once the energy is implanted, the patient will use the energy to heal him or herself by following the thought transfer of abundant health.

The only thing that hinders the use of universal psychic energy in healing is simply the acceptance by humankind of the simple and easy-to-use techniques outlined in this text. Once humankind can better understand how faith, health, and long life are linked, a simpler and healthier lifestyle can be had by everyone in the world.

Only with widespread acceptance of the existence of the use of universal psychic energy will the change come about, as the religious groups will have no choice but to accept the reality that healing is a natural phenomenon. Once this is accepted, humankind can move into a new era of abundant health and mastery of their personal physical body.

In closing, what you have read is a compilation of over 40 years of study in the field of metaphysics, which is on the intangible edge of our physical experience. The information is from many sources, too many to mention and in many cases to remember. This writing is of my experience travelling through the journey of life that we all embarked upon. The ideas have been meticulously worked over until they could be presented in the most basic form that anyone can understand and use. If you notice the lack of technical or mystical jargon, I have succeeded in making the text understandable.

I suggest that you practice the techniques outlined in this book and experience for yourself how the world of energy that we live in works. The energy is out there and waiting for us to use it. Either we will use the energy through subconscious means, or we can consciously take control of the energy about us to have a more glorious life. The choice is ours.

You may not agree with the thoughts that I have put down here, as your experience on the journey in this physical life is most likely much different than the one that I have travelled.

If there is some item in this writing that you do not agree with, search out the reason. You may be one of the individuals with that next vital bit of information that humankind needs to move forward to the evolution of a more powerful existence. My goal in writing this book is not to sway people's opinions on how the universe works, but to share what I learned and to encourage you to think outside of the realm of existence that you are presently in. I challenge you to take that next step out into a greater and more abundant world. I wish you well as you continue your journey through this life.

Ray Kranyak

A fellow traveller through this existence.